QBASE ANAESTHESIA: 4

MCQs FOR THE ANAESTHESIA PRIMARY

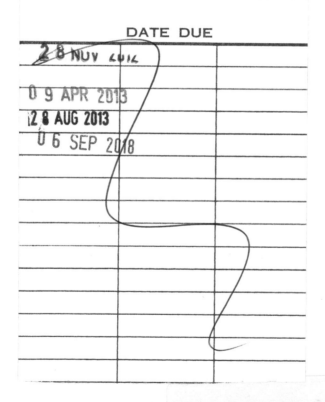

QBASE ANAESTHESIA: 4

MCQs FOR THE ANAESTHESIA PRIMARY

by

Henry G W Paw
BPharm MRPharmS MBBS FRCA
Consultant in Anaesthesia and Intensive Care
York District Hospital

QBase series editors

Edward Hammond MA BM BCh MRCP FRCA
Shackleton Department of Anaesthetics
Southampton University Hospital NHS Trust

Andrew McIndoe MB ChB FRCA
Sir Humphrey Davy Department of Anaesthetics
Bristol Royal Infirmary

GMM

© 1998
Greenwich Medical Media Ltd
219 The Linen Hall
162-168 Regent Street
London
W1R 5TB

ISBN: 1 900151 987
First Published 1998

Distributed worldwide by
Oxford University Press

Designed and Produced by
Diane Parker, Saldatore Limited

Printed in Great Britain by
Ashford Colour Press

CONTENTS

QBase Anaesthesia on CD-ROM

FOREWORD

Multiple Choice Examinations (MCQs) form part of the assessment process in many post-graduate examinations. The MCQ paper is perceived as a threatening test of breadth of knowledge. It is said that the use of negative marking discourages guessing and that candidates fail by answering too many questions. Whilst not a substitute for knowledge and adequate preparation, the assessment ones exam technique can provide valuable feedback leading to improved performance.

Our experience in teaching MCQ technique to candidates suggests that the advice "do not guess" is not correct. Candidates are consistently surprised at the positive benefits of their educated and wild guesses. From a statistical viewpoint, for true random guesses, the negative marking system employed by the Royal College of Anaesthetists tends to produce a null score rather than a negative score. However, with proper preparation, a candidates acquisition of knowledge and insight skews this towards a positive score. This can significantly improve performance leading to success in the examination. QBase has been designed to facilitate the process of assessing exam technique.

This book by Dr Henry Paw provides 300 questions in 5 Primary FRCA papers of 60 questions that complement those in QBase 1 and cover the material required for the examination. The questions are provided with comprehensive explanations and references for further reading. The accompanying CD-ROM contains the latest version of the QBase Interactive MCQ Examination software. It allows the candidate to generate customised exams for revision or assessment purposes. Furthermore the system provides detailed structured analysis of performance and exam technique using the unique "Confidence Option" facility. This CD will update previous versions of QBase.

Candidates for the Primary FRCA Examination should find this book and CD-ROM a valuable learning experience. It should be used repeatedly to improve exam technique. Candidates should remember that knowledge and technique act synergistically to improve scores. Proper preparation will prevent poor performance in the MCQ exam.

Good luck!

Edward Hammond
Andrew McIndoe
QBase Series Developers/Editors
May 1998

EDITORS NOTE

Since we released the first version of QBase, we have tried to respond to the requests and suggestions of trainees on how we can improve it. This latest version of the program contains improvements in the exam analysis functions. These allow you to review you performance based on all the questions in the exam or by subject allowing you to identify areas that need further revision. This also allows you to see whether your technique varies with the subject of the question.

The QBase program resides on your hard disk and reads the data from the QBase CD in your CD drive. If you reinstall QBase from this CD (see back of book for instructions) it will update previous versions of the program. Owners of previous QBase titles will then have the new functions available to them. All QBase CDs will work with the new program. To check for successful installation of the new program, look at the Quick Start Menu screen. It should have 6 exam buttons. Exam 6 will be used by QBase titles containing the appropriate predefined examination 6. The author has included 10 statistics questions on this CD. They do not form part of the current Primary Examination, but candidates may find them useful for revision for the viva and OSCE. They can be accessed via the Exam 6 button or by using the create your own exam option.

Many of you have requested shorter predefined examinations. The exams directory on this CD contains a large number of predefined examinations. To access these exams, go to the main menu screen in the QBase program and select the Resit exam option. From the dialogue box that appears, select the exam directory on your CD drive and then the exam you wish to attempt. The following table gives details of the exams available and their structure. You can save the exam to your hard disk as normal. We have included predefined options to allow you to do all the questions from a subject or a series of 5 mini-exams in each subject that will cover all the questions in each subject in the book without repeating any. We have also included 1 hour mock exams of 30 questions each containing 10 pharmacology, physiology and physics questions. You should allow 40 minutes for exams with 20 questions, 1 hour for exams with 30 questions and 2 hours for exams with 60 questions. To add some spice to your revision, instead of selecting the Resit exam button, we suggest you select the Resit shuffled exam button. The leaves within each question will be shuffled at random, removing your ability to remember the pattern of true/false answers rather than the facts.

We hope that you will find these notes, suggestions and improvements in the program useful in your preparation for the exam. As always, we look forward to your feedback so that we can continue to improve QBase for the future.

Edward Hammond
Andrew McIndoe
QBase Series Developers/Editors
May 1998

Predefined exams included in the exams directory of QBase 4

Exam name	No of Questions	Subjects	Type	Time Allowed
Pharm 1	20	Pharmacology	Revision	40 mins
Pharm 2	20	Pharmacology	Revision	40 mins
Pharm 3	20	Pharmacology	Revision	40 mins
Pharm 4	20	Pharmacology	Reviison	40 mins
Pharm 5	20	Pharmacology	Revision	40 mins
Physiol 1	20	Physiology	Revision	40 mins
Physiol 2	20	Physiology	Revision	40 mins
Physiol 3	20	Physiology	Revision	40 mins
Physiol 4	20	Physiology	Revision	40 mins
Physiol 5	20	Physiology	Revision	40 mins
Physics 1	20	Physics	Revision	40 mins
Physics 2	20	Physics	Revision	40 mins
Physics 3	20	Physics	Revision	40 mins
Physics 4	20	Physics	Revision	40 mins
Physics 5	20	Physics	Revision	40 mins
Exam 11	30	All	Mock	60 mins
Exam 12	30	All	Mock	60 mins
Eaxm 13	30	All	Mock	60 mins
Exam 14	30	All	Mock	60 mins
Exam 15	30	All	Mock	60 mins
Exam 16	30	All	Mock	60 mins
Exam 17	30	All	Mock	60 mins
Exam 18	30	All	Mock	60 mins
Exam 19	30	All	Mock	60 mins
Exam 20	30	All	Mock	60 mins
Pharm 0	100(all questions)	Pharmacology	Revision	200 mins
Physiol 0	100(all questions)	Physiology	Revision	200 mins
Physics 0	100(all questions)	Physics	Revision	200 mins

INTRODUCTION

There is no getting away from MCQ's despite some candidates dislike for them. Unlike essays and vivas which tend to be subjective, MCQs enable an objective test of factual knowledge to be made over a wide area of the syllabus. They are often criticised for being a superficial test, for they do not assess the candidates' ability to weigh up the relative importance of information as may be required in clinical practice.

For certain topics such as physiology, pharmacology, physics and statistics, it is not difficult to set unambiguous MCQs. On the other hand, in clinical anaesthesia and medicine, where things are often less black and white, the setting of questions is more difficult.

A good MCQ can test more than simple factual re-call: reasoning ability and understanding of basic principles can also be assessed. If you strongly disagree with any of the answers given in this book, please do not hesitate to let me know, preferably with the appropriate references.

For the Primary FRCA, the MCQ paper consists of 90 questions to be completed in 3 hours. The paper comprising approximately 30 questions in pharmacology, 30 in physiology and 30 in physics.

MCQs provide a good way of learning: they stimulate interest in a topic which will then encourage further reading. I also believe that the more MCQs you do, the better you become at answering them.

The surest way to pass the MCQs is to have as wider a knowledge as possible of the subjects being tested. Try to identify your weak subjects and concentrate on these.

There is such a thing as 'MCQ technique' and I have, on the following page, listed some pointers which I hope will be useful.

Candidates for the Final FRCA will also benefit from attempting these questions and refreshing their knowledge. It is surprising how much information may have been forgotten in the short interval between the Primary and Final FRCA.

Henry G. W. Paw
Cambridge
May 1998

MCQ TECHNIQUES

Read the question carefully
Each question consists of a stem and five leaves identified by A B C D E. Take care not to let the questions or your answers to one leaf influence your response to the other leaves. Re-read the stem each time in conjunction with the individual leaf as a complete statement.

Trust the examiner
Trust the examiner and do not look for ambiguities and difficulties that do not exist. The questions have all been very carefully selected and vetted. Some candidates read the questions as if they are legal experts and quote obscure references to justify their answer. Take the questions at face value and do not look for difficulties that are not there.

Marking the answer sheet
The answer sheet will be read by an automatic document reader, which transfers the information to a computer marking system. Using the pencil provided mark your answers carefully according to the instructions given. If you then change your mind about the answer, erase your original selection completely with the erasure provided.

There are essentially two ways to mark the sheet. As you go through the questions, you can either mark your answers immediately onto the sheet, or you can mark them in the question book and then transfer to the answer sheet at the end. If you adopt the second approach, you must remember to allow at least 30 mins to transfer the answers from the question book.

Watch the time
Answer only the questions you know in the first round and allow at least 60 mins to go over your answers again and make a reasoned guess at the difficult questions you were unsure about in the first round. At the same time check that you have marked the answer sheet correctly. Do not spend too much time rethinking those answers about which you were originally confident - you might become confused.

To guess or not to guess
True random guesses (i.e. heads or tails) are unlikely to improve your score. As already mentioned in the foreword to this book, the negative marking system employed by the College tends to result in guessing producing a null score. The key is to improve your level of knowledge and skew your guesses towards a positive score. It is probable that the pass mark is around 60% and allowing for a variable proportion of the answers to be wrong, it is unlikely that a candidate will pass if less than 75% of the questions are answered. QBase allows you to assess the benefit of your guesses. You should use the CD repeatedly to determine the strategy that will best reward your knowledge and technique.

ACKNOWLEDGEMENTS

I would like to thank Gavin Smith of Greenwich Medical Media and Dr Edward Hammond for editing this manuscript into electronic format and for their encouragement and support.

Thanks also to Drs Corinna Matt and Peter Bradley who were willing to use the draft copy of this book in their revision for the Primary FRCA and for their valuable comments.

Exam 1

QUESTION 1

Amiodarone may be associated with the following complications

A. Skin discoloration
B. Lung fibrosis
C. Hypothyroidism
D. Shortening of the QT interval
E. Reduction of the serum digoxin level

QUESTION 2

Contra-indicators to ß-blockers include

A. Raynaud's disease
B. Wolff-Parkinson–White syndrome
C. Chronic obstructive pulmonary disease
D. Parkinson's disease
E. Intermittent claudication

QUESTION 3

Digoxin

A. Acts by inhibiting the calcium channel
B. Toxicity is precipitated by hyperkalaemia
C. Must be stopped for 24 hours prior to DC cardioversion
D. Loading dose is highly influenced by renal function
E. Can cause atrial fibrillation

QUESTION 4

Drug combinations that may have significant clinical interaction include

A. Trimethoprim and phenytoin
B. Etomidate and hydrocortisone
C. Rifampicin and propofol
D. Ciprofloxacin and aminophylline
E. Erythromycin and warfarin

QUESTION 5

Regarding the reporting of suspected adverse drug reactions to the committee on safety of medicine (CSM)

A. Only serious reactions to new drugs marked with an inverted black triangle should be reported

B. Cases of well known adverse reactions need not be reported

C. A small payment is made for reporting adverse reactions

D. The therapeutic index is a register of all adverse reactions caused by a drug reported to the CSM

E. Reporting can be made by telephone

QUESTION 6

Remifentanil

A. Undergoes hepatic metabolism

B. Has a half-life of approximately 20 minutes

C. Has a short duration of action because of redistribution

D. Has a potency similar to fentanyl

E. Has a prolonged duration of action in patients with pseudocholinesterase deficiency

QUESTION 7

Verapamil

A. Is structurally related to papaverine

B. Blocks sino–atrial (SA) nodal conduction

C. May be used safely in ventricular arrhythmias

D. Is given in approximately the same dose whether orally or intravenously

E. Is a prodrug

QUESTION 8

Treatment with metformin

A. Is a recognised cause of hypoglycaemia in an elderly diabetic patient

B. Is a recognised cause of diarrhoea

C. Reduces serum triglyceride concentration

D. Increases serum insulin concentration

E. Is contraindicated in the presence of liver disease

QUESTION 9

Pharmacological effects of morphine include

A. Constipation
B. Biliary spasm
C. Histamine release
D. Cough
E. Release of antidiuretic hormone

QUESTION 10

Fentanyl

A. Has a potency 10 times that of morphine
B. Is water-soluble
C. Has a large volume of distribution
D. Does not accumulate even after repeated doses
E. Is metabolised to norfentanyl

QUESTION 11

Diclofenac

A. Works by inhibiting lipo-oxygenase
B. May increase renal blood flow
C. Has antipyretic properties
D. Reversibly promotes platelet aggregation
E. May be used in the last trimester of pregnancy

QUESTION 12

Alfentanil

A. Is more lipid soluble than pethidine
B. Is less lipid soluble than fentanyl
C. Is highly protein bound
D. Is more potent than fentanyl
E. Has clinically important active metabolites

QUESTION 13

Magnesium

A. Has a normal plasma concentration of 0.8-1.2 mmol/litre
B. Is a cerebral vasodilator
C. Has no antiarrhythmic action
D. Is an N-methyl-D-aspartate antagonist
E. Potentiates neuromuscular blockade

QUESTION 14

Tramadol

A. Is a controlled drug
B. Can be administered intravenously
C. Has affinity for binding at the mu opioid receptor comparable to that of morphine
D. Acts predominantly by inhibiting the reuptake of noradrenaline and serotonin (5-HT)
E. May be used concurrently with a MAOI

QUESTION 15

The metabolism of the following observe zero-order kinetics in clinical doses

A. Phenytoin
B. Aspirin
C. Ethanol
D. Propranolol
E. Thiopentone

QUESTION 16

The following are examples of hepatic enzyme inducer

A. Cimetidine
B. Erythromycin
C. Phenytoin
D. Amiodarone
E. Dextropropoxyphene

QUESTION 17

Hepatic first-pass metabolism

A. Is avoided by giving the drug transdermally
B. Is avoided by giving the drug sublingually
C. Is avoided by giving the drug rectally
D. Is avoided by giving an intramuscular injection of the drug
E. Is seen when a drug has a high hepatic extraction ratio

QUESTION 18

The following are characteristics of first-order kinetics

A. A constant proportion of drug metabolised in a given time period
B. The absolute amount eliminated is greatest when plasma concentration is greatest
C. The rate of elimination and elimination half-life is constant, irrespective of plasma concentration
D. The enzyme responsible for the reaction is saturated
E. The reaction is represented by a linear relationship

QUESTION 19

The following are recognised side-effects of digoxin

A. Nausea
B. Xanthopsia
C. Hypokalaemia
D. Hyperuricaemia
E. Gynaecomastia

QUESTION 20

The efficacy of a drug

A. Is greater for drug A if A is effective in a dose of 100 μg than for drug B if B is effective in a dose of 100 mg
B. Is a measure of its therapeutic index
C. Is a measure of the amount of a drug required to produce a given effect
D. Describes the ability of a drug to produce its therapeutic effect
E. Is a measure of the bioavailability of a drug

QUESTION 21

The oxyhaemoglobin dissociation curve is shifted to the right in

A. Pregnancy
B. Cyanide poisoning
C. Carbon monoxide poisoning
D. Fetal haemoglobin
E. Increasing pH

QUESTION 22

The following drugs readily cross the blood-brain barrier

A. Benzylpenicillin
B. Hyoscine hydrobromide
C. Glycopyrollate
D. Atracurium
E. Propofol

QUESTION 23

The following are capable of directly causing pain when applied to nerve endings

A. Prostaglandins
B. Bradykinins
C. Histamine
D. Serotonin (5-HT)
E. Potassium

QUESTION 24

Factors influencing the perception of pain include

A. Anxiety
B. Depression
C. Muscle tension
D. Fatigue
E. Age

QUESTION 25

The following are endocrine consequences of the stress response

A. Decreased ACTH secretion
B. Increased glucagon secretion
C. Increased ADH secretion
D. Increased aldosterone secretion
E. Decreased growth hormone secretion

QUESTION 26

In the third trimester of pregnancy, the following are lowered

A. PaO_2
B. $PaCO_2$
C. Functional residual capacity
D. Vital capacity
E. Lung compliance

QUESTION 27

The following are produced by the adrenal cortex

A. Noradrenaline
B. Dehydroepiandrosterone
C. Angiotensin II
D. Deoxycorticosterone
E. Aldosterone

QUESTION 28

The anterior pituitary gland secretes

A. Oxytocin
B. Thyrotrophin releasing hormone
C. Luteinizing hormone
D. Growth hormone
E. Somatostatin

QUESTION 29

Regarding thyroxine

A. Approximately 80% of circulating thyroxine is bound
B. It is predominantly bound to plasma albumin
C. It is a factor contributing to skeletal growth
D. It decreases the sensitivity of receptors to catecholamines
E. It is a factor affecting the minimum alveolar concentration (MAC) of inhalational anaesthetic agents

QUESTION 30

The pH of the extracellular fluid

A. Is maintained in health between 7.4 and 7.5
B. Is maintained solely by the buffering system of the intra- and extracellular fluids
C. Is increased in hypovolaemic shock
D. Decreases abruptly after a cardiac arrest
E. Influences the binding of drugs to plasma proteins

QUESTION 31

The total cerebral blood flow in normal man is

A. Approximately 15% of the total resting cardiac output
B. Increased significantly by an increase in carbon dioxide concentration in the arterial blood
C. Reduced significantly if the mean systemic BP is reduced from 120 mmHg to 80 mmHg
D. Regulated by sympathetic nerves from the cervical sympathetic chain
E. Increased during intense mental activity

QUESTION 32

In respiratory muscle weakness involving the intercostal muscles and diaphragm

A. The ratio of forced expiratory volume in 1 second (FEV1) to vital capacity (VC) is reduced
B. The ratio of residual volume (RV) to total lung capacity (TLC) is increased
C. Gas transfer that is corrected for lung volume is reduced
D. Hypercapnoea is an early feature
E. The vital capacity (VC) falls when the patient is moved from an upright to a supine position

QUESTION 33

Isovolumetric ventricular contraction of the heart

A. Starts when the aortic valve closes
B. Starts when the mitral valve closes
C. Takes up most of the time the heart spends in ventricular systole
D. Coincides with the 'c' wave in the right atrial pressure trace
E. Coincides with the T wave of the electrocardiogram

QUESTION 34

Regarding the cerebrospinal fluid (CSF)

A. It is a plasma ultrafiltrate
B. The rate of its formation is dependent on the intraventricular pressure over the normal range
C. It has greater buffering capacity than plasma
D. Its main function is in defence against infection
E. It has a similar chloride concentration to plasma

QUESTION 35

In the proximal tubule of the nephron

A. Sodium is actively reabsorbed
B. Bicarbonate is secreted
C. All of the reabsorption of glucose occurs
D. The vast proportion of filtered water is reabsorbed
E. Water reabsorption is under the control of aldosterone

QUESTION 36

Increased urine volume occurs with

A. Glycosuria
B. Increased aldosterone secretion
C. Damage to the posterior pituitary
D. Alcohol consumption
E. Carbonic anhydrase inhibitors

QUESTION 37

Concerning carbon dioxide transport in blood

A. Carbonic anhydrase is present in plasma
B. 25% of carbon dioxide is dissolved
C. 50% is carried as bicarbonate
D. Transport of carbon dioxide is facilitated by deoxygenated haemoglobin
E. Some of the carbon dioxide reacts with haemoglobin to form carbamino compounds

QUESTION 38

Voluntary hyperventilation produces

A. Carpopedal spasm
B. Acidosis
C. Increased cerebral blood flow
D. Peripheral vasodilatation
E. Increased cardiac output

QUESTION 39

The following muscles are responsible for inspiration

A. Internal intercostal muscles
B. External intercostal muscles
C. Diaphragm
D. Muscles of the anterior abdominal wall
E. Sternocleidomastoid

QUESTION 40

There is an increased alveolar–arterial oxygen partial pressure difference (A–a)PO_2 with

A. Hypovolaemia
B. Decreased functional residual capacity
C. Pneumonia
D. Decrease cardiac output
E. Anaesthesia

QUESTION 41

Regarding critical temperature

A. It is the temperature at which a gas exists simultaneously in the gaseous and liquid state at atmospheric pressure
B. The critical temperature of a gas varies with pressure
C. It is the temperature below which, the more a gas is cooled, the less the pressure is required to liquefy it
D. Oxygen at room temperature can be liquefied by 50 bar of pressure
E. Of nitrous oxide is $-116°$ C

QUESTION 42

The following describe Boyle's law

A. The pressure of a gas kept at constant temperature is proportional to its density
B. The pressure of a gas kept at constant temperature varies inversely as the volume
C. For a fixed mass of gas at constant temperature, the product of the pressure and the volume is a constant
D. The volume of a given quantity of gas at constant pressure is directly proportional to the temperature
E. The pressure of a gas kept at constant volume is directly proportional to the temperature

QUESTION 43

The Fluotec 4 vaporiser

A. It delivers a constant vapour concentration from 1 to 15 litres
B. Is protected against back pressure
C. Uses a bellows mechanism for temperature compensation
D. Uses wicks to provide a large surface area for vaporisation
E. If accidentally inverted, will not spill the liquid agent into the bypass

QUESTION 44

The dibucaine test measures the following

A. Activity of acetylcholinesterase
B. Stimulation of pseudocholinesterase activity
C. Inhibition of pseudocholinesterase activity
D. Acetylcholinesterase concentration
E. Susceptibility to malignant hyperthermia

QUESTION 45

Causes of inaccuracies on pulse oximetry include

A. Methaemoglobinaemia
B. Fetal haemoglobin
C. Hypothermia
D. Blue nail polish
E. Extraneous lighting

QUESTION 46

Laminar flow through a tube

A. Is proportional to density
B. Is inversely proportional to viscosity
C. Is inversely proportional to length
D. Is proportional to the square of the radius
E. Is proportional to the pressure drop

QUESTION 47

Pressure

A. Is work per unit time
B. Is force multiplied by distance
C. Is force multiplied by area
D. Can be measured by a column of fluid
E. Is identified by the SI unit, the Newton

QUESTION 48

The following cylinders require reducing valves

A. Oxygen
B. Nitrous oxide
C. Cyclopropane
D. Entonox
E. Carbon dioxide

QUESTION 49

The following statements are true

A. An empty cylinder of oxygen has an absolute pressure of 0 bar
B. A full cylinder of oxygen has a gauge pressure of 137 bar
C. A diver working 10 metres below sea level is at 2 atmospheres absolute pressure
D. Pressure gauges on anaesthetic ventilators usually comprise a simple bellows type of aneroid gauge
E. Pressure gauges on gas cylinders are measured using a Bourdon type of pressure gauge

QUESTION 50

Causes of errors on rotameter reading include

A. Tube not vertical
B. Tube cracked
C. Static electricity
D. Dirt on tube
E. Measuring oxygen on a N_2O rotameter

QUESTION 51

In the measurement of temperature

A. The triple point of water is approximately – 273°C
B. Absolute zero is the temperature at which water exists simultaneously in solid, liquid and gaseous state
C. Electrical resistance increases with rising temperature
D. A thermistor consists of two dissimilar conductors
E. A thermistor relies on the 'Seebeck effect' for its operation

QUESTION 52

One atmosphere of pressure is approximately equivalent to

A. 100 mmHg
B. 10 kPa
C. 100 cm water
D. 14.7 pound per square inch (p.s.i.)
E. 2 atmospheres absolute (ATA)

QUESTION 53

The following statements are true

A. The amount of gas dissolved at any temperature is inversely proportional to its partial pressure
B. The boiling point of a liquid is the temperature at which the saturated vapour pressure equals the ambient atmospheric pressure
C. A solution of 1 osmol/L depresses the boiling point 1.86° C
D. Relative humidity is the actual water vapour pressure as a percentage of the saturated vapour pressure at a given temperature
E. Absolute humidity is the mass of water vapour present in a given volume of gas

QUESTION 54

Concerning laboratory investigations of bleeding disorder

A. Bleeding time is prolonged in haemophilia
B. Prolonged bleeding time occurs with impaired platelet function
C. Activated partial thromboplastin time (APPT) is used to monitor warfarin treatment
D. Activated partial thromboplastin time is sensitive to factors in the intrinsic coagulation pathway
E. Protrombin time (PT) is prolonged in liver failure

QUESTION 55

Entonox

A. In the UK, is stored in blue cylinders with white shoulders
B. The pressure gauge does not give a direct indication of the cylinder content
C. The critical temperature of the mixture is $-116°$ C
D. On cooling the cylinder to a temperature below the critical temperature, separation of the components occur
E. At a temperature below the critical temperature, the initial mixture emitted is richer in oxygen

QUESTION 56

Regarding scavenging

A. The major component of soda lime is sodium hydroxide
B. Passive scavenging systems require a negative pressure relief valve
C. Activated charcoal may be used to absorb nitrous oxide
D. The male connector on scavenging systems has a diameter of 22 mm
E. The female connector on scavenging systems has a diameter of 30 mm

QUESTION 57

An electric current

A. Flows more readily through wet skin than dry skin
B. Is likely to cause muscle contraction when 10 mA is applied externally
C. Is likely to cause arrhythmias when 100 mA is applied externally
D. Is more likely to cause burns when transmitted to a large surface area of the skin
E. Is less likely to be generated in a humid environment

QUESTION   58

Oxygen

A. Is produced commercially by distilling air
B. Is flammable
C. Has a critical temperature of $-36.5°$ C
D. Is stored in the UK in black cylinders with grey shoulders
E. Is stored in the UK in cylinders at a pressure of approximately 50 bar when full

QUESTION   59

Concerning osmolality

A. It depends on the number rather than the type of particles present
B. One mole of sodium chloride dissolved in 1 kg of water has an osmolality of 1 osmol/kg
C. Osmolality of the ECF compartment is greater than that of the ICF compartment due to the greater abundance of sodium
D. Glucose does not contribute to the plasma osmolality
E. Plasma osmolality is approximately 290 mmol/L

QUESTION   60

A rise in temperature

A. Increases the vaporisation rate of volatile agents
B. Decreases the density of fluids
C. Decreases the viscosity of fluid
D. Decreases the viscosity of gases
E. Decreases the osmotic pressure of fluids

Exam 1: Answers

QUESTION 1

A. TRUE   B. TRUE   C. TRUE   D. FALSE   E. FALSE

Dermatological side-effects include slatey grey or blue skin discoloration and photosensitivity. Lung fibrosis is a rare complication of long term, very high dose therapy.

Hyper and hypothyroidism are both possible. Prolongation of QT interval may occur. Amiodarone increases digoxin level by displacement. It may be necessary to reduce the maintenance dosage of digoxin by up to 50% if the patient is also taking amiodarone concurrently.

Ref: W McCaughey, R S J Clarke, J P H Fee, W F M Wallace. Anaesthetic Physiology and Pharmacology, 1st ed. Churchill Livingstone, 1997.

QUESTION 2

A. TRUE   B. FALSE   C. TRUE   D. FALSE   E. TRUE

The three classic groups of patients where ß-blockers are contra-indicated are:-

- Peripheral vascular disease and Raynaud's
- Asthma and COPD
- Heart failure

As well as blockade of ß-receptors, some of these drugs may have additional features such as cardioselectivity, partial agonist activity and membrane-stabilising activity.
Cardioselective ß-blockers such as acebutalol, atenolol, bisoprolol, metoprolol and esmolol block the $ß_1$-receptors to a greater degree than the $ß_2$-receptors.
Some of the ß-blocking drugs e.g. acebutalol and oxprenolol have partial agonist activity, sometimes described as intrinsic sympathomimetic activity (ISA). It has been suggested that drugs with this property have a lower incidence of the undesirable side-effects such as bradycardia, heart failure, cold extremities and bronchospasm.
Propranolol has membrane-stabilising activity, potent local anaesthetic properties and demonstrates class II anti-arrhythmic properties.

Ref: W McCaughey, R S J Clarke, J P H Fee, W F M Wallace. Anaesthetic Physiology and Pharmacology, 1st ed. Churchill Livingstone, 1997.

QUESTION 3

A. FALSE   B. FALSE   C. FALSE   D. FALSE   E. TRUE

Maintenance dose (not loading dose) is highly influenced by renal function. Toxicity is precipitated by hypokalaemia and hypercalaemia. It is not essential to stop digoxin for 24 hours prior to DC cardioversion provided digoxin levels are not in the toxic range. Otherwise there is the risk of unresponsive VF. Digoxin acts on the sodium pump by inhibiting the membrane-bound Na/K ATPase enzyme. This results in accumulation of intracellular sodium and loss of potassium. It works by prolonging AV conduction. Almost any arrhythmia can occur in digox in toxicity including atrial fibrillation.

Ref: W McCaughey, R S J Clarke, J P H Fee, W F M Wallace. Anaesthetic Physiology and Pharmacology, 1st ed. Churchill Livingstone, 1997.

QUESTION 4

A. TRUE B. FALSE C. TRUE D. TRUE E. TRUE

Trimethoprim and phenytoin interfere with folate metabolism causing megaloblastic anaemia. Rifampicin is a liver enzyme inducer which will increase the metabolism of drugs metabolised by the liver. Ciprofloxacin and erythromycin are liver enzyme inhibitors which will decrease the metabolism of drugs metabolised by the liver.

Ref: British National Formulary, 1997

QUESTION 5

A. FALSE B. FALSE C. FALSE D. FALSE E. FALSE

Newer drugs:
These are indicated by the inverted black triangle.
Report all suspected reactions, however minor and irrespective of whether the reaction is well recognised.

Established drugs:
Report all serious suspected reactions even if the effect is well recognised, such as anaphylaxis. There is no need to report well known relatively minor side effects, such as constipation with opioids.

CSM Freephone: for more yellow prepaid lettercards, or advice and information on adverse reactions.

Ref: British National Formulary, 1997

QUESTION 6

A. FALSE B. FALSE C. FALSE D. TRUE E. FALSE

Remifentanil is the latest opioid to be introduced into clinical practice. It does not undergo hepatic metabolism and is unique in that it is broken down by esterases. It has a half-life of approximately 9 minutes and a potency similar to fentanyl. Its duration of action in patients with pseudocholinesterase deficiency is not prolonged.

Ref: Burkle H, Dunbar S, Van Aken H. Remifentanil: A Novel, Short-Acting, mu-opioid. Anesthesia Analgesia 1996; 83: 646-651.

QUESTION 7

A. TRUE B. FALSE C. FALSE D. FALSE E. TRUE

Verapamil is a papaverine derivative. It works by blocking AV nodal conduction. A much smaller dose is required when given IV (oral administration subjected to significant first-pass metabolism). It is dangerous to give verapamil in the presence of ventricular arrhythmias. Verapamil is converted in the body to an active metabolite, norverapamil.

Other prodrugs:-

Parent drug	Active Drug
Carbimazole	Methimazole
Codeine	Morphine
Diamorphine	Monoacetylmorphine and morphine
Enalapril	Enalaprilat
Isosorbide dinitrate	Isosorbide mononitrate
Levodopa	Dopamine
Methyldopa	α-Methyl noradrenaline
Prednisone	Prednisolone
Terfenadine	Fexofenadine

Ref: W McCaughey, R S J Clarke, J P H Fee, W F M Wallace. Anaesthetic Physiology and Pharmacology, 1st ed. Churchill Livingstone, 1997.

QUESTION 8

A. FALSE B. TRUE C. TRUE D. FALSE E. TRUE

Hypoglycaemia is not a problem with metformin, in contrast with the sulphonylureas. Side-effects may be minimised by gradual increase in the dose. Metformin has a beneficial effect on the lipid profile of the diabetic patient. It is commonly given to NIDDMs who are over-weight. Lactic acidosis is rare but may occur in patients with renal or liver failure.

Ref: W McCaughey, R S J Clarke, J P H Fee, W F M Wallace. Anaesthetic Physiology and Pharmacology, 1st ed. Churchill Livingstone, 1997.

QUESTION 9

A. TRUE B. TRUE C. TRUE D. FALSE E. TRUE

Opioids are cough suppressants. Opioids such as codeine, dextromethorphan and pholcodine are ingredients of cough preparations.

Ref: British National Formulary, 1997

QUESTION 10

A. FALSE B. FALSE C. TRUE D. FALSE E. TRUE

Fentanyl is a synthetic opioid related structurally to pethidine. Its analgesic potency is approximately 100 times that of morphine. It is very lipid-soluble and therefore has a large volume of distribution (Vss 375 litres). After repeated doses or infusion there is accumulation. After a single dose, its duration of action is limited to 20-30 minutes due to redistribution. It undergoes hepatic metabolism (N–dealkylation) and is converted to the inactive norfentanyl.

Ref: W McCaughey, R S J Clarke, J P H Fee, W F M Wallace. Anaesthetic Physiology and Pharmacology, 1st ed. Churchill Livingstone, 1997.

QUESTION 11

A. FALSE B. FALSE C. TRUE D. FALSE E. FALSE

Diclofenac, like other non-steroidal anti-inflammatory drugs (NSAIDs), works by inhibiting the cyclo-oxygenase enzyme (not lipo-oxygenase). Prostaglandins are involved in the regulation of renal blood flow and the use of NSAIDs may decrease renal blood flow in susceptible individuals. One of the adverse effects of prostaglandin inhibition is the reversible inhibition of platelet aggregation. Diclofenac is not recommended in pregnancy. Use of NSAIDs may result in premature closure of the ductus arteriosus in the foetus. Low dose aspirin, however, has been used in pregnancy.

Ref: W McCaughey, R S J Clarke, J P H Fee, W F M Wallace. Anaesthetic Physiology and Pharmacology, 1st ed. Churchill Livingstone, 1997.

QUESTION 12

A. TRUE B. TRUE C. TRUE D. FALSE E. FALSE

Alfentanil is more lipid soluble than pethidine, but is less lipid soluble than fentanyl. It is highly protein bound (85-92%) mainly to alpha1-acid glycoprotein. Alfentanil differs from other opioids in having a pKa value below physiological pH (pKa = 6.8). It is between 5 and 10 times less potent than fentanyl. There are no clinically important active metabolites.

Ref: W McCaughey, R S J Clarke, J P H Fee, W F M Wallace. Anaesthetic Physiology and Pharmacology, 1st ed. Churchill Livingstone, 1997.

QUESTION 13

A. TRUE B. TRUE C. FALSE D. TRUE E. TRUE

Magnesium is an N-methyl-D-aspartate antagonist. The normal plasma magnesium concentration ranges between 0.8 and 1.2 mmol/litre. Magnesium is a cerebral vasodilator and has clinically important antiarrhythmic properties. Magnesium potentiates neuromuscular blockade and one of the important signs of magnesium toxicity is muscle weakness.

Ref: H G W Paw, G R Park. Drug Prescribing in Anaesthesia and Intensive Care. 1st ed. Greenwich Medical Media, 1996.

QUESTION 14

A. FALSE B. TRUE C. FALSE D. TRUE E. FALSE

Tramadol is not a controlled drug. It has a weak affinity for opioid receptors. The affinity for binding at the mu receptor is 2.1 µM compared with 0.0003 µM for morphine. Its main mode of action is the modulation of central monoaminergic pathways. As with pethidine (and possibly other opioids), the use of tramadol with MAOI is contraindicated. Both drugs delay the removal of 5-HT from its site of action. The interaction may presents clinically as sudden agitation, unmanageable behaviour, headaches, hypertension or hypotension, rigidity, hyperpyrexia, convulsions and coma.

Ref: Zydol. Searle Drug Information Booklet, 1996.

QUESTION 15

A. TRUE B. TRUE C. TRUE D. FALSE E. FALSE

The metabolism of the following observe zero-order kinetics:

- Phenytoin
- Aspirin
- Ethanol
- Paracetamol (in toxic doses)
- Thiopentone (in toxic doses)

Ref: J W Dundee, R S J Clarke, W McCaughey. Clinical Anaesthetic Pharmacology, 1st ed. Churchill Livingstone, 1991.

QUESTION 16

A. FALSE B. FALSE C. TRUE D. FALSE E. FALSE

Enzyme inducers and inhibitors in clinical use:-

Inducers	Inhibitors
Barbiturates	Amiodarone
Carbamazepine	Cimetidine
Ethanol (chronic)	Ciprofloxacin
Inhalational anaesthetics	Dextropropoxyphene (co-proxamol)
Griseofulvin	Ethanol (acute)
Phenytoin	Etomidate
Primidone	Erythromycin
Rifampicin	Fluconazole
	Ketoconazole
	Metronidazole

Ref: H G W Paw, G R Park. Drug Prescribing in Anaesthesia and Intensive Care, 1st ed. Greenwich Medical Media, 1996.

QUESTION 17

A. TRUE   B. TRUE   C. FALSE   D. TRUE   E. TRUE

Transdermal, sublingual and parenteral (IV, IM, SC) routes avoid the hepatic portal circulation and hence the hepatic first pass metabolism. A variable proportion of the drug given rectally will be absorbed into the portal circulation, therefore first pass metabolism is not totally avoided.

Drugs with high hepatic extraction ratios undergo substantial first pass metabolism.

Ref: W McCaughey, R S J Clarke, J P H Fee, W F M Wallace. Anaesthetic Physiology and Pharmacology, 1st ed. Churchill Livingstone, 1997.

QUESTION 18

A. TRUE   B. TRUE   C. TRUE   D. FALSE   E. FALSE

Zero-order kinetics are observed when the enzyme responsible for the reaction is saturated and when the reaction is represented by a linear relationship.

Summary of the differences between zero-order and first-order kinetics:-

Zero-order:
Absolute amount eliminated is the same, regardless of plasma concentration;
Rate of elimination varies with the plasma concentration;
Constant amount of drug metabolised per unit time;
Reflects saturation of enzyme: occurs when plasma concentration exceeds capacity of enzyme.

First-order:
Constant proportion of drug metabolised in a given time period;
Absolute amount eliminated is greatest when plasma concentration is greatest;
Rate of elimination and elimination half-life are constant, irrespective of concentration.

Ref: J W Dundee, R S J Clarke, W McCaughey. Clinical Anaesthetic Pharmacology, 1st ed. Churchill Livingstone, 1991.

QUESTION 19

A. TRUE   B. TRUE   C. FALSE   D. FALSE   E. TRUE

Xanthopsia is seeing yellow colours. Hypokalaemia predisposes to toxicity but is not a side-effect of digoxin.

Ref: British National Formulary, 1997

QUESTION 20

A. FALSE B. FALSE C. FALSE D. TRUE E. FALSE

The dose of a drug required to produce a given effect decribes its potency, not its efficacy. In the example described, drug A is more potent than drug B.

The therapeutic index of a drug is a measure of its safety (ED50/LD50). Efficacy, however, is a measure of the maximal effect of an agonist.

Ref: W McCaughey, R S J Clarke, J P H Fee, W F M Wallace. Anaesthetic Physiology and Pharmacology, 1st ed. Churchill Livingstone, 1997.

QUESTION 21

A. TRUE B. FALSE C. FALSE D. FALSE E. FALSE

Factors causing a shift of the oxygen dissociation curve:

Left shift:	Right shift:
Fall in temperature	Rise in temperature
Fall in H$^+$ (high pH)	Rise in H$^+$ (low pH)
Fall in red cell 2,3-DPG	Rise in red cell 2,3-DPG
Stored blood	Increase CO_2 tension
Carbon monoxide	Pregnancy★
Fetal haemoglobin	Haemoglobin S
Methaemoglobin	After acclimatisation to altitude

★P50 is higher in normal pregnancy. In PET, the P50 does not increase.

Ref: R D Miller. Anesthesia, 4th ed. Churchill Livingstone, 1994.

QUESTION 22

A. FALSE B. TRUE C. FALSE D. FALSE E. TRUE

Benzylpenicillin does not cross the blood-brain barrier readily unless the meninges are inflamed.
Hyoscine hydrobromide readily crosses the blood-brain barrier.
Hyoscine butylbromide has a quaternary amine group and therefore does not cross the blood-brain barrier as readily.

Ref: J W Dundee, R S J Clarke, W McCaughey. Clinical Anaesthetic Pharmacology, 1st ed. Churchill Livingstone, 1991.

QUESTION 23

A. FALSE B. FALSE C. TRUE D. TRUE E. TRUE

Prostaglandins and bradykinins sensitise the pain fibres to painful stimuli but do not cause pain when directly applied to the nerve endings.

Ref: R D Miller. Anesthesia, 4th ed. Churchill Livingstone, 1994.

QUESTION 24

A. TRUE B. TRUE C. TRUE D. TRUE E. TRUE

Anxiety, depression, muscle tension and fatigue all increase the perception of pain. Increasing age influences the perception of pain depending on ones individual experience.

QUESTION 25

A. FALSE B. TRUE C. TRUE D. TRUE E. FALSE

Endocrine consequences of the stress response

Increased secretion:	Decreased secretion:
ACTH	Insulin
Cortisol	Testosterone
ADH	
Renin	
Aldosterone	
Growth hormone	
Prolactin	
Glucagon	

Ref: W F Ganong. Review of Medical Physiology, 18th ed. Lange, 1997.

QUESTION 26

A. FALSE B. TRUE C. TRUE D. FALSE E. FALSE

There is an increase in minute ventilation (tidal volume increases more than the respiratory rate). Despite the increased CO_2 production, the $PaCO_2$ is reduced from 5 kPa to 4 kPa at term. Because of the greater O_2 consumption and a lowered FRC, there is quicker desaturation when apnoeic. Because of increased alveolar ventilation and the lowered FRC, there is a more rapid uptake of inhalational agent.

Respiratory changes at term:-

Total lung capacity (0); Functional residual capacity (-20%); Residual Volume (-20%); Vital capacity (0); Minute ventilation (+50%); Tidal volume (+40%); Respiratory rate (+15%); Airway resistance (-35%); Lung compliance (0); Chest wall compliance (-45%).

Ref: R D Miller. Anesthesia, 4th ed. Churchill Livingstone, 1994.

QUESTION   27

A. FALSE   B. TRUE   C. FALSE   D. TRUE   E. TRUE

The adrenal cortex produces cortisol, aldosterone, dehydroepiandrosterone and deoxycorti-costerone. Noradrenaline and adrenaline are produced by the adrenal medulla. The conversion of angiotensin I to angiotensin II via angiotensin-converting enzyme (ACE) occurs predom-inantly in the lungs. Angiotensin II acts on the adrenal cortex to increase the secretion of aldosterone.

Ref: W F Ganong. Review of Medical Physiology, 18th ed. Lange, 1997.

QUESTION   28

A. FALSE   B. FALSE   C. TRUE   D. TRUE   E. FALSE

The 6 hormones that are secreted by the anterior pituitary are thyroid stimulating hormone (TSH), adrenocorticotropic hormone (ACTH), luteinising hormone (LH), follicle-stimulating hormone (FSH), prolactin, and growth hormone.
The hormones secreted by the posterior pituitary are oxytocin and vasopressin (ADH). Thyrotrophin releasing hormone and somatostatin (growth hormone- inhibiting hormone) are secreted by the hypothalamus.

Ref: W F Ganong. Review of Medical Physiology, 18th ed. Lange, 1997.

QUESTION   29

A. FALSE   B. FALSE   C. TRUE   D. FALSE   E. TRUE

Normally, 99.98% of circulating thyroxine is bound. Three plasma proteins are responsible for binding thyroxine: albumin, thyroxine-binding prealbumin and thyroxine-binding globulin. Although albumin has the largest capacity to bind thyroxine, the globulins have the greater affinity for thyroxine such that most of the thyroxine is bound to thyroxine-binding globulin. TBG>TBPA>Albumin = 67:20:13.

Hyperthyroidism increases the MAC, whilst hypothyroidism decreases the MAC. Thyroxine increases the sensitivity of receptors to catecholamines.

Ref: W F Ganong. Review of Medical Physiology, 18th ed. Lange, 1997.

QUESTION   30

A. FALSE   B. FALSE   C. FALSE   D. TRUE   E. TRUE

The pH is maintained between 7.35 and 7.42 by the buffering capacity of the bicarbonate/carbonic acid system, the phosphate buffer system and the buffering properties of the serum proteins and haemoglobin. Additional regulation is by the lungs and the kidneys.

Shock and cardiac arrest result in a metabolic acidosis. Due to absence of tissue perfusion, there is a rapid fall in the pH of the extracellular fluid. Binding of drugs to plasma proteins is influenced by the pH of the extracellular fluid.

Ref: W F Ganong. Review of Medical Physiology, 18th ed. Lange, 1997.

QUESTION 31

A. TRUE   B. TRUE   C. FALSE   D. FALSE   E. FALSE

Any substance that increases the acidity of brain tissue will increase cerebral blood flow. Autoregulation of cerebral blood flow between mean arterial pressure limits of 60 mmHg to 140 mmHg is very successful.

The autonomic nervous system plays an insignificant role in the regulation of cerebral blood flow. Regional blood flow is increased during intense mental activity, but the total cerebral blood flow remains constant.

Ref: W F Ganong. Review of Medical Physiology, 18th ed. Lange, 1997.

QUESTION 32

A. FALSE   B. TRUE   C. FALSE   D. FALSE   E. TRUE

Total lung capacity is reduced and residual volume is increased because of the reduction in inspiratory and expiratory capacity. Both of these factors reduce vital capacity but there is no decrease in forced expiratory volume in 1 second suggestive of air flow limitation. The FEV1:VC ratio is normal. Corrected gas transfer is normal. Hypercapnoea is a late feature and usually does not occur until VC has fallen to 50% of normal.

Ref: J B West. Respiratory Physiology - the essentials, 5th ed. Williams and Wilkins, 1995.

QUESTION 33

A. FALSE   B. TRUE   C. FALSE   D. TRUE   E. FALSE

Isovolumetric ventricular contraction of the heart starts when the mitral and tricuspid valves close. This period lasts about 0.05 seconds (25% of ventricular systole), until the pressures in the left and right ventricles exceed the pressures in the aorta and pulmonary artery when the aortic and pulmonary valves open. It coincides with the 'c' wave in the right atrial pressure trace and the QRS complex of the ECG. The 'c' wave results from the tricuspid valve bulging into the right atrium, causing a small but sharp rise in right atrial pressure.

Ref: W F Ganong. Review of Medical Physiology, 18th ed. Lange, 1997.

QUESTION 34

A. TRUE B. FALSE C. FALSE D. FALSE E. FALSE

CSF is an ultrafiltrate of plasma whose composition is modified by transport processes in the endothelial cells of the cerebral capillaries and the choroid epithelium. CSF pressure has no effect on the rate of CSF formation up to pressures well above the normal range. CSF absorption is, however, proportional to the pressure. CSF has a reduced buffering capacity due to its lower protein content when compared to plasma (200 mg/L compared to 6000 mg/L in plasma). The main function of CSF is to act as a 'cushion' to protect the brain. It does not contain any granulocytes or antibodies to defend against infection. The chloride concentration is higher in CSF compared to plasma.

Ref: W F Ganong. Review of Medical Physiology, 18th ed. Lange, 1997.

QUESTION 35

A. TRUE B. FALSE C. TRUE D. TRUE E. FALSE

Na^+ is actively transported out of all parts of the renal tubule except the thin portions of the loop of Henle. Na^+ is pumped into the interstitium by Na^+/K^+ ATPase.

In the proximal tubule, bicarbonate, chloride, glucose and amino acids are reabsorbed along with Na^+ and K^+. Up to 70% of the filtered water is reabsorbed in the proximal tubule. Aldosterone acts mainly in the distal tubule by regulating Na^+ reabsorption. Water then follows passively.

Ref: W F Ganong. Review of Medical Physiology, 18th ed. Lange, 1997.

QUESTION 36

A. TRUE B. FALSE C. TRUE D. TRUE E. TRUE

Glucose is normally completely reabsorbed in the proximal tubule. If the renal threshold for glucose is exceeded and large quantities of glucose remain in the renal tubules, this will exert an appreciable osmotic effect producing an osmotic diuresis. Increased aldosterone secretion results in increased Na^+ (and therefore water) reabsorption. Damage to the posterior pituitary results in lack of ADH producing diabetes insipidus. Alcohol consumption inhibits ADH secretion and therefore increases diuresis. Carbonic anhydrase inhibitors such as acetazolamide are only moderately effective as diuretic agents. They work by decreasing H^+ secretion, with resultant increase in Na^+ and K^+ secretion.

Ref: W F Ganong. Review of Medical Physiology, 18th ed. Lange, 1997.

QUESTION   37

A. FALSE   B. FALSE   C. FALSE   D. TRUE   E. TRUE

The reaction $CO_2 + H_2O \leftrightarrow H_2CO_3$ proceeds slowly unless the enzyme carbonic anhydrase is present. There is no carbonic anhydrase in plasma, but there is an abundant supply in red blood cells. Of the approximately 49 ml of CO_2 in each 100 ml of arterial blood, 2.6 ml (5%) is dissolved, 2.6 ml (5%) is in the form of carbamino compounds and the majority, 43.8 ml (90%) is in HCO_3. Since deoxygenated haemoglobin forms carbamino compounds much more readily than HbO_2, transport of carbon dioxide is facilitated in venous blood.

Ref: A R Aitkenhead, G Smith. Textbook of Anaesthesia, 3rd ed. Churchill Livingstone, 1996.

QUESTION   38

A. TRUE   B. FALSE   C. FALSE   D. FALSE   E. TRUE

Hyperventilation results in hypocapnia and a respiratory alkalosis. As a result of the alkalosis, the plasma ionised calcium level decreases producing the signs of tetany (carpopedal spasm and Chvosteks sign). Cerebral blood flow may be reduced by 30% or more. The cerebral ischaemia causes light-headedness, dizziness and paraesthesia. Hypocapnia has a direct constrictor effect on blood vessels and also increases cardiac output.

Ref: W F Ganong. Review of Medical Physiology, 18th ed. Lange, 1997.

QUESTION   39

A. FALSE   B. TRUE   C. TRUE   D. FALSE   E. TRUE

The diaphragm and the external intercostal muscles are the important muscles during quiet inspiration. The scalene and sternocleidomastoid muscles are accessory inspiratory muscles that help to elevate the thoracic cage during deep laboured respiration. Quiet expiration is passive but the internal intercostals and the muscles of the anterior abdominal wall act as expiratory muscles during forced expiration.

Ref: J B West. Respiratory Physiology - the essentials, 5th ed. Williams and Wilkins, 1995.

QUESTION   40

A. TRUE   B. TRUE   C. TRUE   D. TRUE   E. TRUE

The alveolar-arterial oxygen partial pressure $(A-a)PO_2$ difference is normally about 10 mmHg (1.3 kPa), but may be over 30 mmHg (4 kPa) in the elderly.

There are three major causes of a large $(A-a)PO_2$ gradient:-

- V/Q mismatch
- Diffusion defects
- Anatomical shunt (right to left)

Ref: R S Atkinson, G B Rushman, N J H Davies. Lee's Synopsis of Anaesthesia, 11th ed. Butterworth-Heinemann, 1993.

QUESTION 41

A. FALSE B. FALSE C. TRUE D. FALSE E. FALSE

The critical temperature is different for each gas, but is a constant value for each gas. Provided the temperature is below the critical temperature, the gas can be liquefied by pressure. The critical pressure is that which is required to liquefy a gas at its critical temperature. Above its critical temperature a gas cannot be liquefied however much pressure is applied. Since the critical temperature of oxygen is -116° C, it cannot be liquefied by pressure at room temperature. At -116° C, a pressure of 50 bar is required to liquefy it. The critical temperature of nitrous oxide is 36.5° C and the pressure required to liquefy it at just below this temperature is 74 bar. Below the critical temperature, the more the gas is cooled the less the pressure required to liquefy it. At temperatures lower than the critical temperature the substance may exist as a mixture of both vapour and liquid, depending on its pressure.

Ref: P D Davis, G D Parbrook, G N C Kenny. Basic Physics and Measurement in Anaesthesia, 4th ed. Butterworth-Heinemann, 1995.

QUESTION 42

A. TRUE B. TRUE C. TRUE D. FALSE E. FALSE

Boyle's law can be expressed in the following ways:
   – At a constant temperature, the volume of a mass of gas is inversely proportional to the pressure. Since the density of a gas is inversely proportional to its specific volume, this statement can be reworded:
   – The pressure of a gas kept at constant temperature is proportional to its density
   – The product of the pressure and the specific volume of a gas kept at constant
   temperature is constant.

Charles's law = The volume of a given quantity of gas at constant pressure is directly proportional to the temperature.

Gay-Lussac's law = The pressure of a gas kept at constant volume is directly proportional to the temperature.

Ref: W W Mushin, P L Jones. Physics for the Anaesthetist, 4th ed. Blackwell, 1987.

QUESTION 43

A. FALSE B. TRUE C. FALSE D. TRUE E. TRUE

Back pressure is overcome by the construction of a long inlet tube to the vaporising chamber so that retrograde flow from the vaporiser chamber does not reach the bypass channel. Temperature compensation in the Fluotec 4 vaporiser is acheived by way of a bimetallic strip, which controls the amount of flow through the exit port of the vaporising chamber. The large surface area is provided by a concentric helix, which is bounded by the fabric wicks. If accidentally inverted, the liquid agent will not spill into the bypass. This is one of the new upgrade features from the Fluotec 3 vaporiser.

Ref: A Davey, J T B Moyle, C S Ward. Wards Anaesthetic Equipment, 3rd ed. W B Saunders, 1992.

QUESTION 44

A. FALSE   B. FALSE   C. TRUE   D. FALSE   E. FALSE

Dibucaine number is a measure of the percentage inhibition of the rate of hydrolysis of be zoylcholine in the presence of dibucaine. Dibucaine inhibits the normal pseudocholinesterase enzyme by approximately 80%, but the atypical enzyme remains unaffected.

Atypical cholinesterase

Homozygotes:
- 1 in 3000 of population
- 1-2 hours apnoea
- DN 16-25

Heterozygotes:
- 1 in 25 population
- up to 10 mins apnoea
- DN 50-65

Ref: R S Atkinson, G B Rushman, N J H Davies. Lee's Synopsis of Anaesthesia, 11th ed. Butterworth-Heinemann, 1993.

QUESTION 45

A. TRUE   B. FALSE   C. TRUE   D. TRUE   E. TRUE

Bilirubin causes no significant effect on pulse oximetry. The absorption coefficients for haemoglobin F are no different to those of HbA, so the presence of fetal haemoglobin should not cause an error in pulse oximeter saturation estimates. Pulse oximeters tend to underestimate actual oxygen saturation with significant anaemia. Polycythaemia has no apparent effect upon pulse oximetry reading. Blue nail polish, with absorbance near 660 nm, has the greatest effect on oxygen saturation reading, an artifactual decrease.

Nail varnish, hypothermia, poor perfusion and deeply pigmented skin cause inaccuracies due to weak signals. Increasing concentrations of carboxyhaemoglobin make the pulse oximeter reading tend towards 100%, whereas increasing concentrations of methaemoglobin make the readings tend towards 85%. Other sources of inaccuracies include diathermy interference and extraneous lighting.

Ref: R D Miller. Anesthesia, 4th ed. Churchill Livingstone, 1994.

QUESTION 46

A. FALSE   B. TRUE   C. TRUE   D. FALSE   E. TRUE

Factors that determine laminar flow through a tube are stated by the Hagen-Poiseuille formula:

Flow is proportional to the pressure drop and the radius to the fourth power.
Flow is inversely proportional to viscosity and length.
Density does not affect laminar flow, compared to turbulent flow.

Ref: A R Aitkenhead, G Smith. Textbook of Anaesthesia, 3rd ed. Churchill Livingstone, 1996.

QUESTION 47

A. FALSE B. FALSE C. FALSE D. TRUE E. FALSE

Pressure is force per unit area (F/A).

Pressure is expressed by the SI unit, the Pascal (Pa) = Newtons/square metre

Ref: P D Davis, G D Parbrook, G N C Kenny. Basic Physics and Measurement in Anaesthesia, 4th ed. Butterworth-Heinemann, 1995.

QUESTION 48

A. TRUE B. TRUE C. FALSE D. TRUE E. TRUE

Cyclopropane cylinders do not require a reducing valve.

Pressure at 15°C (bar)	
Oxygen	137
Nitrous oxide	44
Cyclopropane	5
Entonox	137
Carbon dioxide	50

Ref: A Davey, J T B Moyle, C S Ward. Wards Anaesthetic Equipment, 3rd ed. W B Saunders, 1992.

QUESTION 49

A. FALSE B. TRUE C. TRUE D. TRUE E. TRUE

An empty cylinder of oxygen has a gauge pressure of 0 bar but an absolute pressure of about 1 bar (Absolute pressure = gauge pressure + atmospheric pressure).
Lower gas pressures (e.g. on anaesthetic ventilators) are measured using a simple aneroid pressure gauge). High gas pressures (e.g. in medical gas cylinders) are measured using a type of Bourdon gauge.

Ref: P D Davis, G D Parbrook, G N C Kenny. Basic Physics and Measurement in Anaesthesia, 4th ed. Butterworth-Heinemann, 1995.

QUESTION 50

A. TRUE B. TRUE C. TRUE D. TRUE E. TRUE

Static electricity and dirt on the tube or float can cause sticking of the bobbin, especially when low flows are used. The glass tube is slightly smaller on cross-section at the bottom than at the top. Viscosity is important at low flows because gas flow round the bobbin approximates to tubular flow (diameter of orifice less than length), but density is important at high flows (diameter of the orifice greater than length).

Ref: A R Aitkenhead, G Smith. Textbook of Anaesthesia, 3rd ed. Churchill Livingstone, 1996.

QUESTION 51

A. FALSE B. FALSE C. TRUE D. FALSE E. FALSE

The triple point of water is the temperature at which water exists simultaneously in solid, liquid and gaseous state. It is exactly 273.16 K or 0.01° C. The absolute zero is obtained by extrapolation and at this temperature (-273.15° C) an 'ideal' gas would contract and is predicted to occupy zero volume.

The platinum resistance thermometer consists of a length of pure platinum wire. The change in electrical resistance of the wire when its temperature changes is measured with a Wheatstone bridge circuit. Electrical resistance increases with rising temperature (positive temperature coefficient), but this relationship is not linear.

A thermistor, on the other hand, is a semiconductor device, which responds to a rise in temperature by a reduction in electrical resistance (negative temperature coefficient). Seebeck discovered that when two metal conductors of dissimilar materials are connected together at each end to form a circuit, an electromotive force (EMF) is generated which is proportional to the difference in temperatures of the two junctions.

Ref: P D Davis, G D Parbrook, G N C Kenny. Basic Physics and Measurement in Anaesthesia, 4th ed. Butterworth-Heinemann, 1995.

QUESTION 52

A. FALSE B. FALSE C. FALSE D. TRUE E. FALSE

Although the use of SI units is generally accepted in medicine, pressure is still expressed in a variety of units.

1 atmosphere is approximately equivalent to:

1 bar
14.7 p.s.i.
101 kPa
760 mmHg
1000 cmH$_2$O
1 atmospheric absolute (ATA)

Ref: A R Aitkenhead, G Smith. Textbook of Anaesthesia, 3rd ed. Churchill Livingstone, 1996.

QUESTION 53

A. FALSE B. TRUE C. FALSE D. TRUE E. TRUE

Henry's law states that the amount of gas dissolved at any temperature is proportional to its partial pressure. The lower the temperature, the more can dissolve. The boiling point of a liquid is the temperature at which the saturated vapour pressure equals the ambient atmospheric pressure. Osmolarity and osmolality of solutions are measured by the degree to which the freezing (not boiling) point is depressed. A solution of 1 osmol/L depresses the freezing point 1.86° C. Relative humidity is the actual water vapour pressure as a percentage of the saturated vapour pressure at a given temperature. Absolute humidity is the mass of water vapour present in a given volume of gas.

Ref: P D Davis, G D Parbrook, G N C Kenny. Basic Physics and Measurement in Anaesthesia, 4th ed. Butterworth-Heinemann, 1995.

QUESTION 54

A. FALSE B. TRUE C. FALSE D. TRUE E. TRUE

Bleeding time depends on capillary function, as well as platelet numbers and function. It is normally less than 10 minutes. APTT (PTTK) is sensitive to factors in the intrinsic and common pathways. It is used to monitor heparin treatment. The normal APTT is 30-40 seconds.

PT is sensitive to factors in the extrinsic and common pathways. It is used to monitor warfarin treatment and liver function test. Normal PT is 10-14 seconds. Haemophilia A and B have a normal bleeding time and prothrombin time, but prolonged APTT. Von Willebrand's disease has a normal protrombin time, but prolonged bleeding time and APTT.

Ref: A R Aitkenhead, G Smith. Textbook of Anaesthesia, 3rd ed. Churchill Livingstone, 1996.

QUESTION 55

A. FALSE B. FALSE C. FALSE D. TRUE E. TRUE

Entonox is a mixture of 50% oxygen and 50% nitrous oxide. The body of the cylinder is painted blue with the shoulders painted with white/blue quarters. Since the nitrous oxide is in the gaseous state in the cylinder of premixed gases, the pressure gauge gives a direct indication of the cylinder contents. The mixture is compressed into cylinders containing gas at a pressure of 137 bar at 15° C. The nitrous oxide does not liquefy because the presence of oxygen reduces the critical temperature of nitrous oxide. The critical temperature of the mixture is -7°C. Cooling the cylinder to a temperature below -7° C results in separation of liquid nitrous oxide. This results in an initial mixture rich in oxygen, followed by a hypoxic, nitrous oxide rich mixture.

Ref: A Davey, J T B Moyle, C S Ward. Ward's Anaesthetic Equipment, 3rd ed. W B Saunders, 1992.

QUESTION 56

A. FALSE B. TRUE C. FALSE D. FALSE E. TRUE

A major component of soda lime is calcium hydroxide (94%): sodium hydroxide makes up only 5% of the total. Negative pressure (set at -0.5 cmH$_2$O) and positive pressure (set at 10 cmH$_2$O) relief valves must be incorporated in a passive scavenging system to prevent negative or high positive pressures within the system. Activated charcoal placed in the expiratory limb of the breathing system absorbs halogenated volatile agents (not nitrous oxide).

Connectors (male and female) on scavenging systems have a diameter of 30 mm to ensure that inappropriate connections with anaesthetic apparatus cannot be made.

Ref: A Davey, J T B Moyle, C S Ward. Wards Anaesthetic Equipment, 3rd ed. W B Saunders, 1992.

QUESTION   57

A. TRUE   B. FALSE   C. TRUE   D. FALSE   E. FALSE

The frequency adopted in the UK is 50 Hz. A current <1 mA produces no sensation. Tingling sensation occurs at a current of 1 mA. Local pain is produced at 5 mA.
The 'let-go' threshold is variable, but may occur at 15 mA.

Current greater than this 'let-go' threshold will result in greater contraction of flexor to extensor muscles, therefore the victim cannot let go of the source. This 'let-go' threshold varies with the frequency of the current. The frequencies adopted in the UK (50 Hz) and the US (60 Hz) are the most dangerous and has a lower threshold than lower or higher frequencies. Respiratory arrest occurs at 50 mA. Arrhythmias and VF occurs at 80-100 mA. The damage to tissue is related to the current density; a current passing through a small area is more dangerous than the same amount passing through a much larger area.

Sparks are more frequent when the air is dry and the barometric pressure high. Sparks are less likely if the relative humidity is above 60%. The electric current will be generated however, but simply dissipate rather than spark.

Ref: M K Sykes, M D Vickers, C J Hull. Principles of Measurement and Monitoring in Anaesthesia and Intensive Care, 3rd ed. Blackwell, 1991.

QUESTION   58

A. TRUE   B. FALSE   C. FALSE   D. FALSE   E. FALSE

Oxygen is produced commercially by distilling air. Oxygen is tasteless, colourless and odourless. It supports combustion, although the gas itself is not flammable. The critical temperature of oxygen is -119°C. Oxygen cylinders are painted black with white shoulders and are supplied at a pressure of 137 bar at 15°C.

Ref: A R Aitkenhead, G Smith. Textbook of Anaesthesia, 3rd ed. Churchill Livingstone, 1996.

QUESTION   59

A. TRUE   B. FALSE   C. FALSE   D. FALSE   E. FALSE

Osmolality of a solution is determined by the total concentration of dissolved or colloid particles within the solution. It depends on the number rather than the type of particles present. One mole of sodium chloride dissolved in 1 kg of water has an osmolality of 2 osmol/kg, as sodium chloride freely dissociates into the 2 particles, Na and Cl. One mole of urea (which does not dissociate) in 1 kg of water has an osmolality of 1 osmol/kg. The concentration of particles, i.e. the osmolality, within the ICF and the ECF is always equal during equilibrium. Plasma osmolality is approximately 290 mosmol/kg and may be estimated from the formula:

Plasma osmolality (mosmol/kg) = 2[Na] (mmol/L) + Blood glucose (mmol/L) + Blood urea (mmol/L)

Read the question carefully! The units for osmolality are mmol/kg and <u>not</u> mmol/L.

Ref: W F Ganong. Review of Medical Physiology, 18th ed. Lange, 1997.

QUESTION 60

A. TRUE B. TRUE C. TRUE D. FALSE E. FALSE

A rise in temperature:-
- Increases the vaporisation rate of volatile agents, with a higher saturated vapour pressure
- Decreases the density of fluids, due to expansion
- Decreases the viscosity of fluids
- Increases the viscosity of gases, due to increased molecular activity

Exam 2

QUESTION 1

The following drugs readily cross the placenta

A. Physostigmine
B. Glycopyrrolate
C. Naloxone
D. Suxamethonium
E. Heparin

QUESTION 2

In renal impairment

A. Frusemide dosage must be reduced
B. Action of vecuronium is prolonged
C. Drugs bound to plasma proteins are not removed by dialysis
D. Benzylpenicillin may cause convulsions
E. Drugs dependent on renal excretion reach steady state sooner than patients with normal renal function

QUESTION 3

Regarding the ionisation of drugs

A. The pKa of a drug is the pH at which the drug is 100% ionised
B. Drugs with a pKa near physiological pH will show significant changes in the ratio of ionised vs unionised drug
C. The pKa of a drug varies with the pH of the solution
D. A drug with an acid pKa will be mainly unionised in the stomach
E. Local anaesthetics are less effective in an acidic environment

QUESTION 4

The metabolism of morphine involves

A. Acetylation
B. Demethylation
C. Oxidation
D. Methylation
E. Conjugation with glucuronide

QUESTION 5

The total daily dose of the following drugs should be reduced in patients with mild to moderate renal impairment

A. Frusemide
B. Enalapril
C. Ciprofloxacin
D. Erythromycin
E. Metronidazole

QUESTION 6

The cough associated with angiotensin-converting enzyme (ACE) inhibitors

A. Is dose dependent
B. Is more common in men than women
C. Is more common in patients who smoke cigarettes
D. Is more likely to occur when treating hypertension
E. Improves on changing to a different ACE inhibitor

QUESTION 7

Clonidine

A. Is predominantly an α-1 adrenergic agonist
B. Is poorly absorbed orally
C. Lowers the MAC of volatile anaesthetic agents
D. Attenuates the stress response to endotracheal intubation
E. Can be used for spinal analgesia

QUESTION 8

Epileptiform activity may be seen with

A. Propofol
B. Atracurium
C. Neostigmine
D. Etomidate
E. Ketamine

QUESTION 9

The following are acetylcholinesterase inhibitors

A. Malathion
B. Physostigmine
C. Pyridostigmine
D. Edrophonium
E. Ecothiopate

QUESTION 10

The following act as calcium antagonists in smooth muscles

A. Dantrolene
B. Diltiazem
C. Nicardipine
D. Hydralazine
E. Nitroglycerine

QUESTION 11

Factors which may increase the effects of vecuronium include

A. Hypermagnesaemia
B. Hypokalaemia
C. Respiratory acidosis
D. Respiratory alkalosis
E. Hypothermia

QUESTION 12

The minimum alveolar concentration (MAC) of an inhalational agent is reduced in

A. Hypothermia
B. Reduced $PaCO_2$
C. Clonidine
D. Duration of anaesthesia
E. Hypothyroidism

QUESTION 13

The following are metabolised by zero-order kinetics in clinical doses

A. Phenytoin
B. Paracetamol
C. Ethanol
D. Aspirin
E. Thiopentone

QUESTION 14

Sevoflurane

A. Has a higher blood/gas partition coefficient than isoflurane
B. Is more cardiodepressant than isoflurane
C. Has a MAC higher than desflurane
D. Is less pungent than desflurane
E. Has a faster washout than halothane

QUESTION 15

Etomidate

A. Is a phencyclidine derivative
B. Causes more nausea and vomiting than propofol
C. Is rarely associated with anaphylaxis
D. Causes adreno-cortical suppression
E. Is contra-indicated in porphyrias

QUESTION 16

Droperidol

A. Is a phenothiazine
B. Has ß-adrenergic actions
C. Stimulates α receptors
D. Is extensively metabolised by the liver
E. Can cause extrapyramidal side effects

QUESTION 17

Drugs with a prolonged action in the presence of defective plasma acetylcholinesterase include

A. Atracurium
B. Prilocaine
C. Procaine
D. Trimetaphan
E. Esmolol

QUESTION 18

Characteristics of a depolarising block include

A. Initial period of muscle fasciculation
B. Well maintained tetanus during partial block
C. Train-of-four ratio less than 0.75
D. Reversal by anticholinesterases
E. Post-tetanic potentiation

QUESTION 19

The relatively rapid awakening after a single intravenous bolus dose of thiopentone is due to

A. Metabolism by the liver
B. Distribution to fat
C. Distribution to brain, liver and kidneys
D. Elimination in the urine
E. Ester hydrolysis

QUESTION 20

The following are halogenated ethers

A. Halothane
B. Isoflurane
C. Enflurane
D. Desflurane
E. Sevoflurane

QUESTION 21

Concerning the ABO blood groups

A. Type A blood has anti-B antibodies in the plasma
B. Type O blood has no anti-A or anti-B antibodies in the plasma
C. Type O blood can be given to anyone without risk of producing a transfusion reaction
D. The most common blood group is type AB
E. In cross-matching, the donor's plasma is mixed with the recipient's red cells and checked for agglutination

QUESTION 22

The following are anterior pituitary hormones

A. Prolactin
B. Antidiuretic hormone
C. Adrenocorticotrophic hormone
D. Luteinizing hormone
E. Oxytocin

QUESTION 23

The following result in reduced plasma cholinesterase activity

A. Pregnancy
B. Hyperthyroidism
C. Renal failure
D. Nephrotic syndrome
E. Burns

QUESTION 24

The following statements regarding the fluid compartments are true

A. An adult female has a greater percentage of total body water than an adult male
B. The intracellular fluid compartment is approximately 14 litres in a 70 kg man
C. If 5% glucose is infused into a patient it will be equally distributed throughout the fluid compartments
D. If 0.9% saline is infused into a patient it will remain in the extracellular fluid compartment
E. Newborn infants have a greater percentage of body water than adults

QUESTION 25

In pregnancy, the following are normal findings

A. Elevated urea
B. Elevated alkaline phosphates
C. Elevated erythrocyte sedimentation rate (ESR)
D. Raised white cell count
E. Reduced pseudocholinesterase activity

QUESTION 26

The autoregulation of cerebral blood flow

A. Remains constant over a range of systolic blood pressures from 60 to 140 mmHg
B. Curve shows a shift to the left in chronic hypertension
C. Is altered in the acute phase following subarachnoid haemorrhage
D. Is impaired under hypoxic conditions
E. Is impaired in hypercapnia

QUESTION 27

Effects of hypothermia include

A. The presence of a J wave in the ECG
B. A shift of the oxyhaemoglobin dissociation curve to the right
C. Metabolic acidosis
D. A greater solubility of oxygen and carbon dioxide in plasma
E. Impaired coagulation

QUESTION 28

Physiological changes in obesity include

A. A decrease in total body water
B. Increased gastric emptying
C. Increased total lung capacity
D. Increased oxygen consumption
E. Increased in cardiac output

QUESTION 29

Aldosterone secretion is controlled by

A. Plasma sodium concentration
B. Plasma potassium concentration
C. Plasma calcium concentration
D. Adrenocorticotrophic hormone (ACTH)
E. Angiotensin II

QUESTION 30

Renin secretion is controlled by

A. Intrarenal baroreceptors of the efferent arterioles
B. Potassium load reaching the macula densa
C. Renal sympathetic nerve activity
D. Angiotensin
E. ACTH

QUESTION 31

The following statements are true regarding the kidneys

A. There are approximately 1.3 billion nephrons in each kidney
B. They produce aldosterone
C. In a resting state, the kidneys receive 12% of the cardiac output
D. The blood flow in the renal cortex is greater than that in the medulla
E. Autoregulation of renal blood flow occurs

QUESTION 32

Concerning water excretion by the kidneys

A. Over 99% of filtered water is reabsorbed by the kidney
B. Water is actively transported out of the proximal tubule
C. 50% of the filtered water is removed at the end of the proximal tubule
D. The filtered fluid in the distal tubule is hypertonic
E. Antidiuretic hormone decreases the permeability of the collecting duct to water

QUESTION 33

Concerning the withdrawal reflex

A. It is a polysynaptic reflex
B. An example is the knee jerk reflex
C. The sense organ is the muscle spindle
D. As the strength of the stimulus is increased, the reaction time is shortened
E. The response is flexor muscle contraction and inhibition of extensor muscles

QUESTION 34

The following are methods of measuring extracellular fluid volume

A. Labelled albumin
B. Deuterium oxide
C. Labelled inulin
D. Labelled creatinine
E. Labelled glucose

QUESTION 35

Regarding the electrolyte composition of body fluids

A. Cl^- is largely intracellular
B. K^+ is largely intracellular
C. Na^+ is the second most abundant intracellular cation
D. The extracellular fluid has a greater Mg^{2+} concentration than the intracellular space
E. PO_4^{3-} is largely intracellular

QUESTION 36

The following solutions are isotonic

A. 0.9% saline
B. 5% glucose
C. 4% glucose and 0.18% saline
D. Mannitol 10%
E. Hartmann's (compound sodium lactate) solution

QUESTION 37

The chemical mediator released at the following sites is acetylcholine

A. Parasympathetic preganglionic neurones
B. Sympathetic preganglionic neurones
C. Parasympathetic postganglionic neurones
D. Sympathetic postganglionic neurones which innervate sweat glands
E. Sympathetic postganglionic neurones which innervate the heart

QUESTION 38

The following are examples of buffer systems in the body

A. Haemoglobin
B. Glycine
C. Proteins
D. Phosphate
E. Bicarbonate

QUESTION 39

The following statements regarding the anion gap are correct

A. The cations used in the calculation of the anion gap are sodium and potassium
B. The anions used in the calculation of the anion gap are chlorides and phosphates
C. The normal anion gap is between 8 and 10 mmol/l
D. Lactic acidosis causes a metabolic acidosis with a normal anion gap
E. Renal failure causes a metabolic acidosis with a high anion gap

QUESTION 40

The following occur as a response to major surgery

A. Enhanced natriuresis
B. Hyperglycaemia
C. Reduced lipolysis
D. Increased peripheral glucose uptake
E. Potassium retention

QUESTION 41

In the measurement of CVP and PCWP, the following are generally expected

A. Low CVP and a normal PCWP in hypovolaemia
B. High CVP and a normal PCWP in left ventricular failure
C. Normal CVP and high PCWP in pulmonary hypertension
D. High CVP and normal PCWP in tricuspid incompetence
E. High CVP and a normal PCWP in pulmonary embolus

QUESTION 42

Thermodilution cardiac output measurement is inaccurate

A. If the injection is slow (10 ml over 5 seconds)
B. If the injection is erratic
C. If the injectate is at room temperature
D. In the presence of tricuspid regurgitation
E. In the presence of intra–cardiac shunts

QUESTION 43

Gastric intramucosal pH

A. Is calculated using the Bohr equation
B. Values above 7.25 are considered normal
C. Is calculated assuming mucosal bicarbonate is equal to arterial bicarbonate
D. Is lower in splanchnic hypoperfusion
E. Is falsely lowered if air is introduced during sampling

QUESTION 44

Volatile anaesthetic agent concentration may be measured using the following

A. Mass spectrometry
B. Infrared absorption
C. Ultraviolet absorption
D. Polarographic electrode
E. Paramagnetic analyser

QUESTION 45

The following statements regarding transcranial Doppler are true

A. This technique is non-invasive
B. It is most commonly performed through the temporal window
C. It can be performed using the transorbital approach
D. Using transcranial Doppler to estimate cerebral blood flow requires the assumption that the pulse rate is regular
E. It is a sensitive method for detecting cerebral emboli

QUESTION 46

Laser radiation has the following properties

A. It is confined to the invisible portion of the spectrum
B. It is monochromatic
C. It is coherent
D. It is collimated
E. It has a low energy density

QUESTION 47

In magnetic resonance imaging

A. A lead apron needs to be worn by operators
B. The magnetic field created is less than the earth's magnetic field
C. Nickel jewellery will not be attracted by the magnetic field
D. Patients with cardiac pacemakers are contraindicated
E. ECG monitoring may show arrhythmias

QUESTION 48

Electroencephalography (EEG) may be altered by the following

A. Temperature
B. Arterial carbon dioxide tension
C. Hypoxia
D. Uraemia
E. Thiopentone

QUESTION 49

The following measure gas volume

A. Benedict Roth spirometer
B. Vitalograph
C. Wright respirometer
D. Fleisch pneumotachograph
E. Rotameter

QUESTION 50

The following are measured directly in a blood gas analyser

A. Oxygen saturation
B. Oxygen tension
C. Carbon dioxide tension
D. Hydrogen ion concentration
E. Bicarbonate concentration

QUESTION 51

The following parameters are needed to determine the anatomical dead space in Fowler's method

A. Arterial oxygen tension
B. Inspired oxygen tension
C. Inspired carbon dioxide tension
D. Expired carbon dioxide tension
E. Nitrogen analysis of expired air

QUESTION 52

The following parameters are needed to determine the physiological dead space in Bohr's method

A. Tidal volume
B. Respiratory rate
C. Arterial oxygen tension
D. Inspired oxygen tension
E. Alveolar carbon dioxide tension

QUESTION 53

The percentage of oxygen in the alveolar air

A. Depends on the atmospheric pressure
B. Depends on the ambient humidity
C. May be increased by giving supplementary oxygen
D. May be increased during induction of anaesthesia with a mixture of 21% oxygen in nitrous oxide
E. Is greater than the mixed expired air

QUESTION 54

Soda lime in the anaesthetic circuit

A. Is mainly composed of sodium carbonate
B. Needs moisture to absorb carbon dioxide
C. Gets hot in use
D. Can be used to absorb nitrous oxide
E. Produces carbon monoxide if dry

QUESTION 55

A volatile anaesthetic agent has a SVP of 243 mmHg. If the total fresh gas flow is 5 l/min of which 200 ml/min is directed through the vaporising chamber, the inspired conc. will be approximately

A. 0.25%
B. 0.5%
C. 1.0%
D. 1.5%
E. 2.0%

QUESTION 56

Concerning the relationship between end-tidal CO$_2$ and PaCO$_2$

A. In healthy lungs the $P_{ET}CO_2$ is approximately 0.5 kPa greater than the PaCO$_2$
B. $P_{ET}CO_2$ and PaCO$_2$ difference is reduced when ventilated with larger tidal volumes
C. $P_{ET}CO_2$ and PaCO$_2$ difference is reduced in pregnancy
D. A reduction in pulmonary blood flow by 50% would produce approximately a 50% reduction in $P_{ET}CO_2$
E. In COPD, the $P_{ET}CO_2$ and PaCO$_2$ difference can be reduced by reducing ventilator frequency and increasing tidal volume

QUESTION 57

The Magill circuit in spontaneous ventilation

A. Is an example of a Mapleson A circuit
B. Requires the fresh gas flow rate to equal the patient's minute volume ventilation to prevent rebreathing
C. Can be made more efficient by placement of the expiratory valve close to the reservoir bag
D. Improves its rebreathing characteristics if the length of tubing is doubled
E. Is suitable for children weighing over 15 kg

QUESTION 58

The saturated vapour pressure of a liquid

A. Is the pressure exerted at the critical temperature
B. Increases with increase temperature
C. Is directly proportional to the atmospheric pressure
D. Is equal to atmospheric pressure at its boiling point
E. Can be greater than its boiling point

QUESTION 59

The following techniques may be used to monitor cerebral function during carotid endarterectomy

A. Somatosensory evoked potentials
B. Transcranial Doppler
C. Cerebral oximetry
D. Carotid stump pressure
E. Conjunctival oxygen tension

QUESTION 60

When taking blood pressure with a sphygmomanometer, a falsely high reading may result from

A. Using a standard cuff on an obese person
B. Using too narrow a cuff
C. Letting the cuff down slowly
D. Arteriosclerosis
E. Placement of the sphygmomanometer above the level of the heart

Exam 2: Answers

QUESTION 1

A. TRUE B. FALSE C. TRUE D. FALSE E. FALSE

Physostigmine, being a tertiary amine, readily crosses the placenta. Glycopyrrolate is a quarternary ammonium compound and is highly ionized, thus making membrane penetration difficult. Naloxone, because of its high lipid solubility, is easily transferred to the foetus and can be administered to the mother to counteract anticipated respiratory depression in the infant. Suxamethonium and heparin are highly ionized and threfore do not readily cross the placenta.

Ref: W McCaughey, R S J Clarke, J P H Fee, W F M Wallace. Anaesthetic Physiology and Pharmacology, 1st ed. Churchill Livingstone, 1997.

QUESTION 2

A. FALSE B. TRUE C. TRUE D. TRUE E. FALSE

Higher doses of frusemide are needed although the risk of toxicity is increased. Benzylpenicillin is predominantly excreted by the kidneys, therefore higher levels are reached in renal failure.

Ref: W McCaughey, R S J Clarke, J P H Fee, W F M Wallace. Anaesthetic Physiology and Pharmacology, 1st ed. Churchill Livingstone, 1997.

QUESTION 3

A. FALSE B. TRUE C. FALSE D. TRUE E. TRUE

The pKa of a drug is the pH at which the drug is 50% ionised. Due to the steepness of the graph, drugs with a pKa near physiological pH will show significant changes in the percentage of drug that is ionised versus unionised. The pKa is a constant for each drug. The stomach has a very low pH and a drug with an acid pKa such as aspirin (pKa 3.5), will be mainly unionised, and thus will be readily absorbed across the gastric membrane.

Local anaesthetics are weak bases, and in an acidic environment (localised infection, acidotic or poorly perfused tissues) where the pH is below the pKa, the ionised form predominates and thus crosses the neural membrane less readily.

Ref: W McCaughey, R S J Clarke, J P H Fee, W F M Wallace. Anaesthetic Physiology and Pharmacology, 1st ed. Churchill Livingstone, 1997.

QUESTION 4

A. FALSE B. TRUE C. TRUE D. TRUE E. TRUE

Morphine metabolism involves demethylation, oxidation, conjugation with glucuronide, and methylation to codeine.

Ref: J W Dundee, R S J Clarke, W McCaughey. Clinical Anaesthetic Pharmacology, 1st ed. Churchill Livingstone, 1991.

QUESTION 5

A. FALSE B. TRUE C. TRUE D. FALSE E. FALSE

Ciprofloxacin and enalapril undergo significant renal excretion. Although frusemide is potentially nephrotoxic, it is necessary to increase the dose in renal impairment to produce the same effect. The main route of excretion for erythromycin and metronidazole is hepatic.

Ref: British National Formulary, 1997

QUESTION 6

A. FALSE B. FALSE C. FALSE D. FALSE E. FALSE

A dry, tickly, non-productive cough has been reported in up to 15% of patients treated with ACE inhibitors. The incidence of ACE inhibitor-induced cough is twice as common in women as in men, but there is no difference between smokers and non-smokers, or in patients being treated for hypertension or heart failure

Changing to a different ACE inhibitor is unlikely to have a significant effect on the cough. There is no evidence of dose dependency. Withdrawal of the offending drug leads to complete recovery within days. Recurrence occurs on rechallenge.

Ref: Prescribers Journal. 31(4), 1991.

QUESTION 7

A. FALSE B. FALSE C. TRUE D. TRUE E. TRUE

Clonidine is an α-2 adrenergic agonist whose action is predominantly central. The ratio of $\alpha2:\alpha1$ activity is 200:1. The analgesic action of clonidine is exerted centrally, although the precise site and mechanism are uncertain. It is also effective when administered via the intrathecal and epidural routes. Clonidine results in a reduction in anaesthetic agent requirements by up to 50%. Clonidine attenuates the increase in blood pressure and heart rate in response to stressful stimuli (laryngoscopy, endotracheal intubation, skin incision).

Clonidine is rapidly and almost completely absorbed when given orally, reaching a peak plasma level within 60-90 mins.

Ref: W McCaughey, R S J Clarke, J P H Fee, W F M Wallace. Anaesthetic Physiology and Pharmacology, 1st ed. Churchill Livingstone, 1997.

QUESTION 8

A. TRUE   B. FALSE   C. FALSE   D. TRUE   E. FALSE

There is now no doubt that propofol can cause epileptic fits in those who are susceptible and may be delayed after stopping its administration. In addition, propofol has anti-convulsant action, although this is less marked than that of thiopentone. It has been shown to inhibit electroconvulsive therapy (ECT) convulsions and has been used to suppress convulsions in a variety of conditions, some of them refractory to barbiturates and phenytoin.

One of the breakdown products of atracurium, laudanosine (but not atracurium per se) has been shown to cause fits in dogs above a threshold of 17 µg/ml. In humans, the threshold for fits has not been established. Neostigmine does not cross the blood brain barrier. Rare cases of fits have been reported with etomidate. Ketamine is not epileptogenic but enhanced skeletal muscle tone may be manifested by tonic and clonic movements sometimes resembling fits.

Ref: W McCaughey, R S J Clarke, J P H Fee, W F M Wallace. Anaesthetic Physiology and Pharmacology, 1st ed. Churchill Livingstone, 1997.

QUESTION 9

A. TRUE   B. TRUE   C. TRUE   D. TRUE   E. TRUE

Malathion is a constituent of some headlice shampoos and is also used in sheepdips. Edrophonium is used in the diagnosis of myasthenia gravis (the tensilon test). Physostigmine is used in the treatment of myasthenia gravis. Physostigmine and ecothiopate eyedrops are used as miotics in the treatment of glaucoma. Donepezil (Aricept), another inhibitor of acetyl-cholinesterase, is the first specific drug for treating Alzheimer's disease.

Ref: W McCaughey, R S J Clarke, J P H Fee, W F M Wallace. Anaesthetic Physiology and Pharmacology, 1st ed. Churchill Livingstone, 1997.

QUESTION 10

A. FALSE   B. TRUE   C. TRUE   D. FALSE   E. FALSE

Dantrolene is a direct-acting skeletal muscle relaxant. It uncouples the excitation-contraction process by inhibiting the release of ionised calcium from the terminal cisternae of the sarcoplasmic reticulum into the sarcoplasm. It does not act on smooth muscles and has no action on the neuromuscular junction. Diltiazem and nicardipine are calcium-channel blockers acting on myocardial cells, conducting system of the heart, and cells of the vascular smooth muscle. Hydralazine and nitroglycerine are both vasodilators but not calcium antagonists.

Ref: W McCaughey, R S J Clarke, J P H Fee, W F M Wallace. Anaesthetic Physiology and Pharmacology, 1st ed. Churchill Livingstone, 1997.

QUESTION 11

A. TRUE B. TRUE C. TRUE D. FALSE E. TRUE

Factors which may increase the effects of vecuronium are: Hypermagnesaemia, hypokalaemia, hypocalcaemia, hypoproteinaemia, dehydration, acidosis, hypercapnoea, cachexia, hypothermia, prior use of suxamethonium, and concurrent use of aminoglycoside antibiotics, α-adrenergic blocking agents, ß-adrenergic blocking agents and MAO inhibiting agents.

Ref: W McCaughey, R S J Clarke, J P H Fee, W F M Wallace. Anaesthetic Physiology and Pharmacology, 1st ed. Churchill Livingstone, 1997.

QUESTION 12

A. TRUE B. FALSE C. TRUE D. FALSE E. TRUE

Factors affecting the MAC.

Decrease MAC:
Age, benzodiazepines, opioids, nitrous oxide, neuromuscular blockers, alpha-2 agonists, hypothermia, severe hypotension, hypoxaemia, hypothyroidism, pregnancy, increase atmospheric pressure, chronic use of amphetamine

Increase MAC:
Hyperthermia, hyperthyroidism, acute usage of amphetamine

No change:
Sex, hypercarbia, hypocarbia, duration of anaesthesia

Ref: R D Miller. Anesthesia, 4th ed. Churchill Livingstone, 1994.

QUESTION 13

A. TRUE B. FALSE C. TRUE D. TRUE E. FALSE

Paracetamol and barbiturates are metabolised by zero-order kinetics only in toxic doses.

Ref: J W Dundee, R S J Clarke, W McCaughey. Clinical Anaesthetic Pharmacology, 1st ed. Churchill Livingstone, 1991.

QUESTION 14

A. FALSE B. FALSE C. FALSE D. TRUE E. TRUE

Sevoflurane has a lower blood /gas partition coefficient than isoflurane (0.6 vs 1.4). It does not sensitise the myocardium to catecholamines and has relatively little effect on the cardiovascular system. The MAC of sevofluarane is approximately 2% compared to 6% for desflurane. It is less pungent than desflurane and is therefore suitable for inhalational induction. Because of the lower blood/gas and oil/gas partition coefficients, sevoflurane has a faster washout than halothane.

Ref: A R Aitkenhead, G Smith. Textbook of Anaesthesia, 3rd ed. Churchill Livingstone, 1996.

QUESTION 15

A. FALSE   B. TRUE   C. TRUE   D. TRUE   E. TRUE

Etomidate is a carboxylated imidazole. Ketamine is a phencyclidine derivative. The incidence of nausea and vomiting is very much higher than propofol. Allergic reactions are extremely rare (1 in 450,000). Etomidate causes adreno-corticol suppression even after a single bolus dose. Etomidate is contraindicated in porphyrias.

Ref: W McCaughey, R S J Clarke, J P H Fee, W F M Wallace. Anaesthetic Physiology and Pharmacology, 1st ed. Churchill Livingstone, 1997.

QUESTION 16

A. FALSE   B. FALSE   C. FALSE   D. TRUE   E. TRUE

Droperidol is a butyrophenone and it acts by interfering with dopaminergic transmission in the brain. Because it blocks dopamine receptors, it may cause extrapyramidal side effects. In addition, it blocks the α-adrenergic receptors but has no effect on the ß-adrenergic receptors. It is extensively metabolised by the liver.

Ref: W McCaughey, R S J Clarke, J P H Fee, W F M Wallace. Anaesthetic Physiology and Pharmacology, 1st ed. Churchill Livingstone, 1997.

QUESTION 17

A. FALSE   B. FALSE   C. TRUE   D. TRUE   E. FALSE

Suxamethonium, mivacurium, procaine and trimetaphan are broken down by plasma acetyl-cholinesterase and a prolonged action may be expected in the presence of defective acetyl-cholinesterase enzyme. Esmolol is broken down by non-specific esterases.

Ref: W McCaughey, R S J Clarke, J P H Fee, W F M Wallace. Anaesthetic Physiology and Pharmacology, 1st ed. Churchill Livingstone, 1997.

QUESTION 18

A. TRUE   B. TRUE   C. FALSE   D. FALSE   E. FALSE

Characteristics of a depolarising block include:

- Initial period of muscle fasciculation
- Well maintained tetanus with no fade

- An absence of post–tetanic potentiation
- Anticholinesterases may potentiate the block

Ref: A R Aitkenhead, G Smith. Textbook of Anaesthesia, 3rd ed. Churchill Livingstone, 1996.

QUESTION 19

A. FALSE   B. FALSE   C. TRUE   D. FALSE   E. FALSE

The mechanism responsible for the relatively rapid awakening after a single i.v. bolus dose of thiopentone is the redistribution into well-perfused organs (brain, liver and kidneys). Despite the high lipid solubility of thiopentone, fat contributes little to the initial redistribution or termination of its action because of the poor blood supply.

Ref: A R Aitkenhead, G Smith. Textbook of Anaesthesia, 3rd ed. Churchill Livingstone, 1996.

QUESTION 20

A. FALSE   B. TRUE   C. TRUE   D. TRUE   E. TRUE

Halothane is a halogenated hydrocarbon ($CF_3CHClBr$).

Ref: A R Aitkenhead, G Smith. Textbook of Anaesthesia, 3rd ed. Churchill Livingstone, 1996.

QUESTION 21

A. TRUE   B. FALSE   C. FALSE   D. FALSE   E. FALSE

Type A blood has anti–B antibodies in the plasma. Type O blood has both anti–A and anti–B antibodies in the plasma. Individuals with type O blood are 'universal donors', and type O blood can be given to anyone without producing a transfusion reaction due to ABO incompatibility. However, the possibilities of reaction due to incompatibilities other than ABO incompatibilities always exists. The most common blood group is type O. In cross-matching, the donor's red cells are mixed with the recipient's plasma and checked for agglutination.

Ref: W F Ganong. Review of Medical Physiology, 18th ed. Lange, 1997.

QUESTION 22

A. TRUE   B. FALSE   C. TRUE   D. TRUE   E. FALSE

The anterior pituitary secretes 6 hormones: ACTH, TSH, FSH, LH, growth hormone and prolactin. Antidiuretic hormone and oxytocin are both secreted by the posterior pituitary.

Ref: W F Ganong. Review of Medical Physiology, 18th ed. Lange, 1997.

QUESTION   23

A. TRUE   B. FALSE   C. TRUE   D. FALSE   E. TRUE
Causes of altered plasma cholinesterase activity:-

Decrease activity	Increase activity
Pregnancy	Hyperthyroidism
Malignancy	Nephrotic syndrome
Malnutrition	Mental retardation
Hepatic failure	Depression
Heart failure	Hyperlipidaemia
Renal failure	Obesity
Hypothyroidism	
Burns	

Ref: L Davis, J J Britten, M Morgan. Cholinesterase: its significance in anaesthetic practice. Anaesthesia 1997; 52: 244-260.

QUESTION   24

A. FALSE   B. FALSE   C. TRUE   D. TRUE   E. TRUE

Adult males are roughly 60% water and adult females 55%. Females have a greater proportion of body fat than males. The average 70 kg male contains 42 litres of water (60ml/kg), and two-thirds of this is intracellular fluid (ICF). The remaining one-third is extracellular (ECF) and is divided between the interstitial fluid and the vascular compartments. A fourth ('transcellular') compartment includes cerebrospinal, synovial, pleural and pericardial fluids, plus water in the gut. Normally the latter represents a small proportion of the total, but in disease (e.g. in para-lytic ileus or massive pleural effusion), it can become important. Newborn infants comprise some 75% water. The proportion of water decreases with increasing age. All infused Na^+ remains in the ECF; Na^+ cannot gain access to the ICF because of the sodium pump. As 0.9% saline is isotonic, there is no change in ECF osmolality and therefore no water exchange occurs across the cell membrane.

Ref: A R Aitkenhead, G Smith. Textbook of Anaesthesia, 3rd ed. Churchill Livingstone, 1996.

QUESTION   25

A. FALSE   B. TRUE   C. TRUE   D. TRUE   E. TRUE

The raised white cell count is due mainly to neutrophil leucocytosis. Pseudocholinesterase activity is decreased by up to 30% but this does not prolong the action of suxamethonium to a clinically significant extent.

Ref: A R Aitkenhead, G Smith. Textbook of Anaesthesia, 3rd ed. Churchill Livingstone, 1996.

QUESTION 26

A. FALSE   B. FALSE   C. TRUE   D. TRUE   E. TRUE

Cerebral blood flow remains constant over a range of mean systemic (not systolic!) blood pressures from 60 to 140 mmHg. Above and below these mean blood pressures, cerebral blood flow is increased and decreased respectively. In chronic hypertension, the autoregulation curve is shifted to the right. Autoregulation is lost around areas of intracerebral pathology. Autoregulation is impaired by hypoxia and hypercapnia. Cerebral blood flow increases when the PaO_2 decreases to 6.7 kPa (50 mmHg) and is doubled at a PaO_2 of 4 kPa (30 mmHg).

Ref: A R Aitkenhead, G Smith. Textbook of Anaesthesia, 3rd ed. Churchill Livingstone, 1996.

QUESTION 27

A. TRUE   B. FALSE   C. TRUE   D. TRUE   E. TRUE

Other ECG changes associated with hypothermia include prolongation of the P-R interval, widened QRS complex, increased Q-T interval and S-T elevation. The oxyhaemoglobin dissociation curve shifts to the left thus reducing oxygen availability to the tissues. The clotting mechanisms are depressed and there is a fall in platelet count.

Ref: R S Atkinson, G B Rushman, N J H Davies. Lee's Synopsis of Anaesthesia, 11th ed. Butterworth-Heinemann, 1993.

QUESTION 28

A. TRUE   B. FALSE   C. FALSE   D. TRUE   E. TRUE

The volume of distribution of drugs may be altered significantly by a decrease in total body water and an increase in body fat. The incidence of hiatus hernia is increased in the obese and this, together with a rise in intra-abdominal pressure and delayed gastric emptying, puts them at greater risk of aspiration of gastric contents under anaesthesia. Changes in lung volume include a decrease in functional residual capacity, total lung capacity, inspiratory capacity, vital capacity and expiratory reserve volume, whilst residual volume remains unchanged. Obese patients have increased oxygen consumption and carbon dioxide production. They have an increased blood volume and cardiac output proportional to their oxygen demand

Ref: R D Miller. Anesthesia, 4th ed. Churchill Livingstone, 1994.

QUESTION 29

A. TRUE   B. TRUE   C. FALSE   D. TRUE   E. TRUE

Aldosterone secretion is controlled by 4 main factors:-

- Plasma sodium concentration
- Plasma potassium concentration

- ACTH
- Angiotensin II

An increase in plasma sodium concentration inhibits the release of aldosterone to favour salt loss, while increased plasma potassium stimulates aldosterone release. An increase in circulatory ACTH, as in trauma, also stimulates the release of aldosterone. These three factors are of lesser importance than the fourth – the plasma concentration of angiotensin II.

Ref: W F Ganong. Review of Medical Physiology, 18th ed. Lange, 1997.

QUESTION 30

A. FALSE   B. FALSE   C. TRUE   D. TRUE   E. FALSE

Renin secretion is controlled by:-

- Intrarenal baroreceptors of the afferent (not efferent) arterioles
- Sodium or possibly chloride ions (not potassium) in the macula densa
- Renal sympathetic nerve activity
- Angiotensin

A fall in the arteriolar pressure in the afferent arterioles and decreased sodium load reaching the macula densa both stimulate release of renin from the juxta-glomerular apparatus. Renal sympathetic nerve activity causes constriction of the afferent arterioles to give reduced pressure distal to the constriction and therefore stimulation of the intrarenal baroreceptors to promote renin release. The glomerular filtration rate (GFR) is therefore lowered and the sodium load reaching the macula densa will consequently decrease. Sympathetic activity thus stimulates renin release indirectly by means of the first two controlling factors, in addition to direct stimulation of the beta–adrenergic receptors in the renin-secreting granular cells. Angiotensin itself exerts a direct negative feedback on renin release and therefore on its own production.

Ref: W F Ganong. Review of Medical Physiology, 18th ed. Lange, 1997.

QUESTION 31

A. FALSE   B. FALSE   C. FALSE   D. TRUE   E. TRUE

There are approximately 1.3 million nephrons in each kidney. Aldosterone is produced by the adrenal cortex. The kidneys produce prostaglandins, kinins, renin and 1,25–dihydroxychole-calciferol. In a resting state, the kidneys receive 1.2 L of blood per minute, which is approximately 25% of the cardiac output. The blood flow in the renal cortex is estimated to be at least 20 times greater than that in the medulla. Renal autoregulation of renal blood flow is present even in denervated and in isolated, perfused kidneys.

Ref: W F Ganong. Review of Medical Physiology, 18th ed. Lange, 1997.

QUESTION 32

A. TRUE   B. FALSE   C. FALSE   D. FALSE   E. FALSE

Normally, 180 litres of fluid is filtered through the glomeruli each day with 179 litres reabsorbed, producing 1 litre urine per day on average. The transport of water is a passive one: i.e. water moves passively along the osmotic gradients set up by active transport of solutes. Up to 70% of the filtered water is removed by the time the filtrate reaches the end of the proximal tubule. The filtered tubular fluid in the distal tubule is hypotonic. ADH from the posterior pituitary gland increases the permeability of the collecting duct to water.

Percentage of filtered water removed at various parts of the nephron:-

Proximal tubule	60-70%
Loop of Henlé	15%
Distal tubule	5%
Collecting ducts	10%

Changes in the osmolality of tubular fluid in various parts of the nephron:-

Proximal tubule	Isotonic
Descending limb of the loop of Henlé	Hypertonic
Ascending limb of the loop of Henlé	Hypotonic
Distal tubule	More hypotonic
Collecting ducts	Hypertonic

Ref: W F Ganong. Review of Medical Physiology, 18th ed. Lange, 1997.

QUESTION 33

A. TRUE   B. FALSE   C. FALSE   D. TRUE   E. TRUE

The withdrawal reflex is a polysynaptic reflex that occurs in response to a painful stimulus. The response is flexor muscle contraction and inhibition of extensor muscles, so that the part stimulated is flexed and withdrawn from the stimulus. As the strength of the stimulus is increased, the reaction time is shortened.

The knee jerk is a monosynaptic reflex. The stimulus is stretch of the muscle, and the response is contraction of the muscle being stretched. The sense organ in this case is the muscle spindle.

Ref: W F Ganong. Review of Medical Physiology, 18th ed. Lange, 1997.

QUESTION 34

A. FALSE   B. FALSE   C. TRUE   D. FALSE   E. FALSE

The extracellular fluid volume is difficult to measure because the limits of this space are ill defined and lymph cannot be separated from the ECF and is measured with it. Inulin, mannitol and sucrose have been used to measure ECF volume. Albumin labelled with radioactive iodine or dyes (Evans blue) that are bound to plasma protein can be used to measure plasma volume. Deuterium oxide (heavy water) is used to measure total body water.

Ref: W F Ganong. Review of Medical Physiology, 18th ed. Lange, 1997.

QUESTION 35

A. FALSE   B. TRUE   C. FALSE   D. FALSE   E. TRUE

Na^+ and Cl^- are largely extracellular, whereas K^+ and PO_4^{3-} are largely intracellular. Mg^{2+} is the fourth most plentiful cation and second most abundant intracellular cation (99% of which is intracellular).

Ref: W F Ganong. Review of Medical Physiology, 18th ed. Lange, 1997.

QUESTION 36

A. TRUE   B. TRUE   C. TRUE   D. FALSE   E. TRUE

Solutions that have the same osmolality as plasma are said to be isotonic. The following solutions are isotonic: 0.9% saline, 5% glucose, 4% glucose + 0.18% saline, and Hartmann's (Ringer's lactate) solution. Mannitol 10% and 20% are hypertonic. 5% glucose solution is isotonic when initially infused intravenously, but the glucose is metabolised, so the net effect is that of infusing a hypotonic solution.

Ref: A R Aitkenhead, G Smith. Textbook of Anaesthesia, 3rd ed. Churchill Livingstone, 1996.

QUESTION 37

A. TRUE   B. TRUE   C. TRUE   D. TRUE   E. FALSE

The cholinergic neurones are:-

- All preganglionic neurones.
- Parasympathetic postganglionic neurones.
- Sympathetic postganglionic neurones which innervate sweat glands.
- Sympathetic postganglionic neurones which end on blood vessels in skeletal muscles and produce vasodilatation when stimulated.

The remaining postganglionic sympathetic neurones are noradrenergic.

Ref: W F Ganong. Review of Medical Physiology, 18th ed. Lange, 1997.

QUESTION 38

A. TRUE   B. FALSE   C. TRUE   D. TRUE   E. TRUE

Compartment distribution of the main buffer systems in the body:-

Interstitial fluid:	Bicarbonate
Plasma:	Bicarbonate Proteins Inorganic phosphate
Red blood cells:	Bicarbonate Haemoglobin Inorganic phosphate Organic phosphate 2,3-DPG

Ref: W F Ganong. Review of Medical Physiology, 18th ed. Lange, 1997.

QUESTION   39

A. TRUE   B. FALSE   C. FALSE   D. FALSE   E. TRUE

The cations used in the calculation of the anion gap are sodium and potassium. The anions used in the calculation of the anion gap are chlorides and bicarbonates.

Anion gap = $(Na^+ + K^+) - (Cl^- + HCO_3^-)$

The normal anion gap is between 10 and 18 mmol/l.

The most useful application of the anion gap is in classifying metabolic acidosis into two types.
Metabolic acidosis with high anion gap:-
- Renal failure
- Lactic acidosis
- Ketoacidosis
- Poisoning with aspirin, methanol, ethylene glycol, and paraldehyde

Metabolic acidosis with normal anion gap:-
- Diarrhoea
- Ureterosigmoidostomy
- Renal tubular acidosis
- Treatment with carbonic anhydrase inhibitors

Ref: A R Aitkenhead, G Smith. Textbook of Anaesthesia, 3rd ed. Churchill Livingstone, 1996.

QUESTION   40

A. FALSE   B. TRUE   C. FALSE   D. FALSE   E. FALSE

The stress response results in

- Sodium and water retention
- Potassium loss
- Increased protein breakdown
- Decreased protein synthesis
- Increased gluconeogenesis

- Increased glycogenolysis
- Decreased peripheral glucose uptake
- Increased lipolysis
- Decreased lipogenesis

Ref: W F Ganong. Review of Medical Physiology, 18th ed. Lange, 1997.

QUESTION 41

A. FALSE   B. FALSE   C. FALSE   D. TRUE   E. TRUE

CVP	PCWP	Causes
Increased	Normal	Right Ventricular Failure Pulmonary Embolus Pulmonary Hypertension Tricuspid Incompetence
Decreased	Decreased	Hypovolaemia
Normal	Increased	Left Ventricular Failure
Increased	Increased	Congestive Heart Failure Hypervolaemia

QUESTION 42

A. TRUE   B. TRUE   C. FALSE   D. TRUE   E. TRUE

It is not necessary to use iced injectate in the thermodilution cardiac output measurement, as long as there is a temperature difference between the injectate and blood temperature. Warmer solutions require higher thermistor sensitivities than do iced solutions. Use of iced solutions increases the signal-to-noise ratio.

Each injection should be timed to occur at the same point in the respiratory cycle to assure comparability of measurements. Patients on mechanical ventilation should have the injection made at the end of expiration.

The injection should be made as rapidly and as smoothly as possible to create a smooth thermodilution curve. Most computation constants assume injection in less than 4 seconds. Any factors such as valvular lesion or intra-cardiac shunt that might decrease intraventricular mixing or result in streaming of blood/indicator will result in an over or underestimation of cardiac output.

Ref: C Scurr, S Feldman, N Soni. Scientific Foundations of Anaesthesia, 4th ed. Heinemann, 1990.

QUESTION 43

A. FALSE   B. FALSE   C. TRUE   D. TRUE   E. FALSE

The gastric intramucosal pH (pHi) is an indirect estimation of the pH of the superficial mucosal cells of the stomach wall. It is calculated using the Henderson-Hasselbach equation. A low value reflects the inability of the oxygen supply to meet the metabolic demands of these tissues. The pHi is considered normal if values are above 7.35. In splanchnic hypoperfusion pHi will be low. The value will be falsely raised if air is introduced during sampling. Studies have shown the potential usefulness of pHi in identifying critically ill patients at risk of poor outcome, as a therapeutic endpoint and guide to adequate resuscitation.

Ref: M G Mythen, A R Webb. The Role of Gut Mucosal Hypoperfusion in the Pathogenesis of Postoperative Organ Dysfunction. Intensive Care Medicine 1994; 20: 203-209.

QUESTION 44

A. TRUE   B. TRUE   C. TRUE   D. FALSE   E. FALSE

Volatile anaesthetic agent concentration may be measured using mass spectrometry, infrared absorption and ultraviolet absorption. Polarographic and paramagnetic analysers measure oxygen concentration.

Ref: C Scurr, S Feldman, N Soni. Scientific Foundations of Anaesthesia, 4th ed. Heinemann, 1990.

QUESTION 45

A. TRUE   B. TRUE   C. TRUE   D. FALSE   E. TRUE

Transcranial Doppler is most commonly performed through the temporal window, where the skull is relatively thin, but can be performed using the transorbital, suboccipital or submandibular approaches.

Using transcranial Doppler to estimate cerebral blood flow requires the assumption that the cross-sectional area of the insonated vessel and the viscosity of the blood flowing through the vessel remain constant.

Ref: K S Drader, I A Herrick. Carotid endarterctomy: Monitoring and its Effect on Outcome. Anesthesiology Clinics of North America 1997; 15: 613-629.

QUESTION 46

A. FALSE   B. TRUE   C. TRUE   D. TRUE   E. FALSE

Laser is an acronym for 'light amplification by stimulated emission of radiation'. The radiation may be in the visible or the invisible infrared part of the spectrum.

It has the following properties:-

- Monochromatic: all the photons have the same energy, wavelength, and frequency
- Coherent: all the photons are in phase
- Collimated: the beam does not diverge
- High energy density: a large amount of energy is concentrated in a small area

Ref: M Sosis. Anesthesia for Laser Surgery. International Anesthesiology Clinics 1990; 2(2): 119-131.

QUESTION 47

A. FALSE   B. FALSE   C. FALSE   D. TRUE   E. TRUE

Ionising radiation is not used in MRI and lead aprons are therefore not required. The magnetic field created is up to 2 teslas. The earth's magnetic field is only 0.00005 teslas or 40,000 times less. Ferromagnetic metals (iron, nickel, cobalt) will be attracted by he magnetic field.

Ref: R D Miller. Anesthesia, 4th ed. Churchill Livingstone, 1994.

QUESTION 48

A. TRUE   B. TRUE   C. TRUE   D. TRUE   E. TRUE

The EEG reflects the spontaneous electrical activity of cortical pyramidal neurones arising from inhibitory and excitatory postsynaptic potentials. The EEG may be altered by a large number of physiological factors, including temperature, arterial carbon dioxide tension, hypoxaemia, and electrolyte abnormalities. Anaesthetic drugs also affect EEG morphology, depending on the drugs used and the depth of anaesthesia.

Ref: K S Drader, I A Herrick. Carotid endarterctomy: Monitoring and its Effect on Outcome. Anesthesiology Clinics of North America 1997; 15: 613-629.

QUESTION 49

A. TRUE   B. TRUE   C. TRUE   D. FALSE   E. FALSE

The Benedict Roth spirometer, Vitalograph and Wright respirometer all measure gas volume. The Fleisch pneumotachograph and the Rotameter both measure flow.

Ref: P D Davis, G D Parbrook, G N C Kenny. Basic Physics and Measurement in Anaesthesia, 4th ed. Butterworth-Heinemann, 1995.

QUESTION 50

A. FALSE   B. TRUE   C. TRUE   D. TRUE   E. FALSE

Oxygen, carbon dioxide and hydrogen ion concentrations are measured directly in a blood gas analyser. Oxygen saturation, bicarbonate concentration and the base excess are derived values.

QUESTION 51

A. FALSE   B. FALSE   C. FALSE   D. FALSE   E. TRUE

Fowler's method is used to measure the anatomical dead space. 100% oxygen is inspired at the end of a normal inspiration so that the dead space is filled with oxygen. The partial pressure of nitrogen is measured on expiration. It is initially zero, rising to a plateau as the supplemental oxygen is washed out. The volume of air expired at the mid point of the initial rising phase of nitrogen concentration represents the volume of the dead space.

Ref: J B West. Respiratory Physiology - the essentials, 5th ed. Williams and Wilkins, 1995.

QUESTION 52

A. TRUE   B. FALSE   C. FALSE   D. FALSE   E. TRUE

Bohr's method measures the volume of the lung which does not eliminate carbon dioxide (physiological dead space). In normal subjects, the physiological dead space and anatomical dead space are very nearly the same. In patients with lung disease, however, the physiological dead space may be considerably larger because of ventilation/perfusion (V/Q) inequalities with the lung.

Bohr's equation can be written as:-

$$\frac{V_D}{V_T} = \frac{P_A CO_2 - P_E CO_2}{P_A CO_2}$$

Where V_D = physiological dead space; V_T = tidal volume; $P_A CO_2$ = alveolar CO_2; $P_E CO_2$ = mixed expired CO_2.

The PCO_2 in alveolar gas and arterial blood ($PaCO_2$) is virtually identical so that the equation is often written as:-

$$\frac{V_D}{V_T} = \frac{PaCO_2 - P_E CO_2}{PaCO_2}$$

Ref: J B West. Respiratory Physiology - the essentials, 5th ed. Williams and Wilkins, 1995.

QUESTION 53

A. FALSE   B. FALSE   C. TRUE   D. TRUE   E. FALSE

Whatever the outside air humidity, the nose is such an efficient humidifier that air drawn into the respiratory tract becomes fully saturated in the alveoli at 37° C. The concentration of water is constant at 44 mg/l which represents a fractional concentration of 6.2%. Oxygen supplementation will increase the fractional inspired oxygen and therefore the alveolar percentage.

Because nitrous oxide is approximately 30 times more soluble in blood than nitrogen, the alveolar gas volume is effectively reduced. Since the amount of oxygen remains the same, an increase in the percentage of oxygen results. Expired air is a mixture of alveolar and dead space gas, which therefore has a higher percentage of oxygen than alveolar air.

Ref: A R Aitkenhead, G Smith. Textbook of Anaesthesia, 3rd ed. Churchill Livingstone, 1996.

QUESTION 54

A. FALSE B. TRUE C. TRUE D. FALSE E. TRUE

Soda lime is approximately 94% calcium hydroxide. As it absorbs carbon dioxide, heat and moisture are produced. Soda lime does not absorb nitrous oxide or volatile anaesthetic agents. Barium hydroxide (Baralyme) produces significantly more carbon monoxide than soda lime when dry. In the UK, baralyme is not available, and anaesthetic machines in current use do not have fresh gas flow placed upstream of the absorbent canister, which causes the absorbent to become excessively dry.

Ref: A R Aitkenhead, G Smith. Textbook of Anaesthesia, 3rd ed. Churchill Livingstone, 1996.

QUESTION 55

A. FALSE B. FALSE C. FALSE D. FALSE E. TRUE

Plenum vaporisers work on the principle that the part of the flow that goes through the vaporising chamber becomes fully saturated. Since the SVP is 243 mmHg, fresh gas passing through the vaporising chamber will have a vapour concentration approximately one-third of the atmospheric pressure (760 mmHg). Thus 200 ml of fresh gas passing through the vaporising chamber will have 100 ml of vapour added to it. The final vapour concentration is therefore 100 ml in 5000 ml which is approximately 2%.

Note: If you ever get a question like this and you cannot work out the answer, it is best to answer all questions as false. You will then get a score of at least 3, instead of zero by not answering the question at all.

Ref: P D Davis, G D Parbrook, G N C Kenny. Basic Physics and Measurement in Anaesthesia, 4th ed. Butterworth-Heinemann, 1995.

QUESTION 56

A. FALSE B. TRUE C. TRUE D. TRUE E. TRUE

A sample of end-tidal gas is assumed to have come from the alveoli where it is in equilibrium with pulmonary capillary blood. End-tidal CO_2 is therefore usually taken to be an indirect measure of arterial CO_2, and in adults with healthy lungs, the $P_{ET}CO_2$ is approximately 0.3-0.6 kPa less than the $PaCO_2$. Following a pulmonary embolus in a previously healthy lung, there is a sudden increase in alveolar dead space because all lung units are ventilated but only some are perfused. Since all these lung units empty at the same rate, there is a constant dilution of the CO_2 from the perfused alveoli by the non-CO_2 containing gas from the unperfused alveoli. Theoretically, a reduction in pulmonary blood flow by 50% would produce a 50% reduction in $P_{ET}CO_2$. In COPD, there is widespread V/Q mismatching throughout the lung. A $P_{ET}CO_2$ - $PaCO_2$ difference of over 2 kPa is not unusual. Reducing the frequency (to allow more time for equilibration) and increasing the tidal volume (to maximise the perfusing of dependent lung segments) of ventilation minimises this difference.

Ref: M Harwick, P Hutton. Capnography: Fundamentals of Current Clinical Practice. Current Anaesthesia and Critical Care 1990; 1: 176-180.

QUESTION 57

A. TRUE   B. FALSE   C. FALSE   D. FALSE   E. FALSE

If the system is functioning correctly and no leaks are present, a fresh gas flow rate equal to the patients alveolar (not minute volume) ventilation is sufficient to prevent rebreathing during spontaneous ventilation. In practice, a slightly higher fresh gas flow rate is selected in order to compensate for leaks.

None of the modifications indicated will improve the efficiency of Magill's original system.

Due to the large dead space it is not suitable for children weighing less than 25 kg.

Ref: A R Aitkenhead, G Smith. Textbook of Anaesthesia, 3rd ed. Churchill Livingstone, 1996.

QUESTION 58

A. FALSE   B. TRUE   C. FALSE   D. TRUE   E. FALSE

The vapour pressure of a liquid depends only on the physical properties of the liquid and the temperature. It does not depend on the barometric pressure within the range of pressures encountered in anaesthesia.

The saturated vapour pressure (SVP) occurs when as many molecules are leaving the liquid phase to escape to the vapour phase as are returning. The SVP of a liquid is equal to the atmospheric pressure at its boiling point.

Ref: A R Aitkenhead, G Smith. Textbook of Anaesthesia, 3rd ed. Churchill Livingstone, 1996.

QUESTION 59

A. TRUE   B. TRUE   C. TRUE   D. TRUE   E. TRUE

Ref: K S Drader, I A Herrick. Carotid endarterctomy: Monitoring and its Effect on Outcome. Anesthesiology Clinics of North America 1997; 15: 613-629.

QUESTION 60

A. TRUE   B. TRUE   C. FALSE   D. FALSE   E. FALSE

The width of the cuff is important – too narrow a cuff gives too high a reading, and too wide a cuff may give too low a reading. The WHO recommends a cuff 14 cm wide for an average adult. As a rough guide, the cuff should cover approximatey two-thirds of the upper arm or its width should be about 20% greater than the diameter of the arm. Arteriosclerotic arteries may produce a high systolic blood pressure, but this is not falsely high. When compared to direct methods, indirect measurements tend to overestimate at lower pressures and underestimate at higher pressures.

Ref: M K Sykes, M D Vickers, C J Hull. Principles of Measurement and Monitoring in Anaesthesia and Intensive Care, 3rd ed. Blackwell, 1991.

Exam 3

QUESTION 1

The following drugs may be given via an endotracheal tube

A. Adrenaline
B. Atropine
C. Lignocaine
D. Sodium bicarbonate
E. Calcium chloride

QUESTION 2

Aminophylline

A. Is a phosphodiesterase inhibitor
B. Is a mixture of theophylline and ethylenediamine
C. Has a wide therapeutic index
D. Dosage requirements are increased in smokers
E. May be given intramuscularly

QUESTION 3

Adenosine

A. Is effective in ventricular tachycardia
B. Has a half life of approximately 10 minutes
C. Should be given as a slow intravenous bolus
D. Can result in wheezing
E. Causes coronary vasodilatation

QUESTION 4

Nitric oxide

A. Was formerly known as endothelium-derived relaxing factor
B. Causes pulmonary vasodilatation
C. Inhibits platelet aggregation
D. When released into the circulation, results in rapid deactivation
E. Should be administered in combination with oxygen

QUESTION 5

Dopexamine

A. Is a precursor of noradrenaline
B. Exerts its predominant effect by stimulating ß-1 adrenoceptors
C. Is a weak ß-2 adrenoceptor agonist
D. Reduces atrial filling pressures
E. Produces pulmonary hypertension

QUESTION 6

The following drug interactions are synergistic

A. Propofol and midazolam
B. Propofol and ketamine
C. Propofol and thiopentone
D. Thiopentone and midazolam
E. Propofol and alfentanil

QUESTION 7

The following drugs may be used as antidotes for the treatment of the associated overdoses or poisonings

A. Naloxone and co-proxamol overdose
B. Methionine and paracetamol overdose
C. Sodium calciumedetate and cyanide poisoning
D. Desferrioxime and lead poisoning
E. Pralidoxime mesylate and organophosphorus poisoning

QUESTION 8

The following drugs exhibit significant hepatic first-pass metabolism

A. Aspirin
B. Morphine
C. Propranolol
D. Glyceryl trinitrate
E. Alcohol

QUESTION 9

The following are positive inotropes

A. Verapamil
B. Enoximone
C. Propranolol
D. Amiodarone
E. Theophylline

QUESTION 10

Isoflurane

A. Is a fluorinated hydrocarbon
B. Has a MAC of 0.5% in 70% nitrous oxide
C. Causes less respiratory depression than halothane
D. Should not be used with soda lime
E. Has a greater oil/gas partition coefficient than enflurane

QUESTION 11

Atropine

A. Is more sedative than hyoscine
B. Reverses the miosis caused by opioids
C. Inhibits sweating
D. Readily crosses the blood-brain barrier
E. Causes hyperpyrexia in overdose

QUESTION 12

The minimum alveolar concentration (MAC) of an inhalational anaesthetic agent

A. Is an index of anaesthetic potency
B. Is proportional to lipid solubility
C. Is determined in subjects premedicated with omnopon and scopolamine
D. Decreases with increasing duration of anaesthesia
E. Can be determined by frequent blood sampling

QUESTION 13

Drugs with greater than 50% oral bioavailability include

A. Morphine
B. Propranolol
C. Methadone
D. Atenolol
E. Gentamicin

QUESTION 14

The following drugs readily cross the blood–brain barrier

A. Physostigmine
B. Neostigmine
C. Dopamine
D. Propranolol
E. Glycopyrollate

QUESTION 15

Metabolism of the following drugs are affected by the acetylator status of the individual

A. Hydralazine
B. Isoniazid
C. Propranolol
D. Amiodarone
E. Digoxin

QUESTION 16

The following drugs are excreted mostly unchanged by the kidneys

A. Digoxin
B. Gentamicin
C. Theophylline
D. Morphine
E. Vecuronium

QUESTION 17

Adverse effects of amitriptyline overdose include

A. Dilated pupils
B. Cardiac arrhythmias
C. Convulsion
D. Hyperreflexia
E. Metabolic acidosis

QUESTION 18

Protein binding is affected by

A. pH
B. Age
C. Renal disease
D. Liver disease
E. Pregnancy

QUESTION 19

Drugs of use in ventricular extrasystole include

A. Verapamil
B. Mexiletine
C. Amiodarone
D. Flecainide
E. Digoxin

QUESTION 20

The following statements are true

A. In drug intoxication, haemodialysis is more likely to lower plasma concentration of the drug if its volume of distribution is large
B. The half-life of a drug is the time taken for the clinical effect to be reduced by half
C. Intravenously administered drug has 100% bioavailability
D. Efficacy is the ability of the drug to bind to the receptor site
E. Drugs with long half-life require a loading dose to achieve a rapid therapeutic concentration

QUESTION 21

The following statements are correct

A. There is approximately 50% greater resistance to breathing through the nose than through the mouth
B. Total airway resistance is greater in the small airways than the trachea
C. Type I pneumocytes contain distinctive lamellar vacuoles
D. Type I pneumocytes secrete and store surfactant
E. The pores of Kohn are holes in the alveolar wall

QUESTION 22

Respiratory physiology in the neonate, compared with the adult, shows

A. Lower lung compliance
B. Higher airway resistance
C. Almost entirely diaphragmatic ventilation
D. Higher physiological dead space
E. Higher respiratory rate

QUESTION 23

Foetal haemoglobin

A. Forms approximately 80% of haemoglobin at birth
B. Is made up of two alpha and two delta chains
C. Forms approximately 20% of haemoglobin at the age of 6 months
D. Has a lower affinity for oxygen than adult haemoglobin (HbA)
E. Is present in ß-thalassaemia major

QUESTION 24

ECG changes in hypokalaemia include

A. Reduced P wave
B. Widened QRS complex
C. Shortened QT interval
D. Reduced height of T wave
E. Increased height of U wave

QUESTION 25

Lung surfactant

A. Contains mucopolysaccharides
B. Increases surface tension
C. Production is decreased when lung blood flow to that region of the lung is stopped
D. Increases compliance
E. Makes the pressure in connected alveoli identical

QUESTION 26

Functional residual capacity

A. Increases with obesity
B. Increases with anaesthesia
C. Decreases with age
D. Can be measured by a Helium dilution technique
E. Causes regional hypoventilation when less than the closing capacity

QUESTION 27

Regarding the composition of the cerebrospinal fluid

A. The PO_2 is the same as that of arterial blood
B. The pH is lower than arterial blood
C. The protein level is higher than venous blood
D. The glucose level is lower than venous blood
E. The chloride level is higher than venous blood

QUESTION 28

The following statements are correct regarding arterial blood at 30°C compared with 37°C

A. Lower PO_2
B. Lower PCO_2
C. Increase in pH
D. Decrease in HCO_3^-
E. Lower oxygen saturation

QUESTION 29

Gastric emptying is delayed by

A. Fat in the duodenum
B. Acid in the duodenum
C. Stress
D. Volume of fluid
E. Atropine

QUESTION 30

Concerning lung volumes and capacities

A. The total volume of both lungs is the vital capacity
B. The sum of the resting tidal volume and the inspiratory reserve volume is the inspiratory capacity
C. The volume which may be forcibly exhaled in 1 sec is greater than 85% of the vital capacity
D. The functional residual capacity can be measured with the spirometer
E. The sum of the inspiratory reserve volume and the expiratory reserve volume is the vital capacity

QUESTION 31

Concerning coronary blood flow

A. It is approximately 20% of the cardiac output at rest
B. It is highest during systole
C. It is reduced during hypoxia
D. Increased myocardial oxygen demand results in increased oxygen extraction but little increase in coronary blood flow
E. It is reduced in aortic stenosis

QUESTION 32

During quiet respiration in a healthy human subject

A. The diaphragm contracts during inspiration
B. Alveolar pressure is sub-atmospheric during expiration
C. Intrapleural pressure is sub-atmospheric throughout the respiratory cycle
D. The volume of gas exhaled per minute is less than 12 litres
E. Dead space ventilation is approximately equal to alveolar ventilation

QUESTION 33

Regarding the ventricular action potential

A. The rapid phase of depolarisation is due to sodium influx
B. The plateau phase is due to a sustained increase in membrane sodium permeability
C. Repolarisation is associated with an increase in membrane permeability to potassium
D. The absolute refractory period last for approximately 1 millisecond
E. The refractory period is almost as long as the muscle twitch which it elicits

QUESTION 34

Cardiac excitation in the normal heart

A. Is initiated spontaneously in the sino-atrial (SA) node
B. Takes 0.2 ms to be transmitted through the atrium to the atrioventricular (AV) node
C. Is transmitted most slowly at the atrioventricular (AV) node
D. Is conducted down the interventricular septum in a single tract of conducting tissue – the bundle of His
E. Spreads from the endocardial to the epicardial surface of the ventricle at a rate of about 0.3 m/s

QUESTION 35

The speed of onset of inhalational anaesthesia depends on

A. Blood/gas solubility
B. Lipid solubility
C. Cardiac output
D. Inspired concentration
E. Pulmonary blood flow

QUESTION 36

Potassium

A. Concentration in the plasma is a good reflection of total body potassium
B. In the plasma rises in metabolic acidosis
C. Enters cells in the presence of insulin
D. Is excreted in the presence of aldosterone
E. Is depleted by nasogastric suctioning

QUESTION 37

The following are used in calculating the oxygen content of arterial blood

A. Haemoglobin concentration
B. Cardiac output
C. Arterial oxygen saturation
D. Arterial oxygen tension (PaO_2)
E. Mixed venous oxygen saturation (SvO_2)

QUESTION 38

The electroencephalogram (EEG)

A. Records brain wave potential in the range 3-5 mV
B. Contains alpha waves in a restful subject with open eyes
C. Produces a characteristic 3 Hz spike pattern in grand mal fits
D. Is predominantly comprised of delta waves in an alert subject
E. Is generally flat during anaesthesia

QUESTION 39

In the peripheral nervous system

A. Myelinated neurones are devoid of myelin at the nodes of Ranvier
B. Schawnn cells form myelin sheaths around the myelinated neurones
C. Unmyelinated neurones do not contain Schwann cells
D. Nodes of Ranvier are absent in unmyelinated neurones
E. The autonomic postganglionic neurones are mostly unmyelinated C fibres

QUESTION 40

Concerning the autonomic nervous system

A. Sympathetic preganglionic cell bodies lie in the inter-mediolateral columns of the spinal cord between segments T1 to L3
B. Stimulation of the sympathetic innervation of the bronchial smooth muscle causes bronchodilatation
C. Stimulation of the sympathetic innervation of the stomach causes imhibition of gastric secretion
D. All preganglionic sympathetic neurones synapse in paravertebral ganglia
E. There are no discrete parasympathetic ganglia

QUESTION 41

The following gases can be measured using infrared analysers

A. Oxygen
B. Nitrous oxide
C. Nitrogen
D. Carbon dioxide
E. Sevoflurane

QUESTION 42

Wright's respirometer

A. Is a pneumotachograph
B. Over-reads at high flows
C. Under-reads at low flow
D. Gives slightly higher readings with mixtures of nitrous oxide and oxygen than for air
E. Should ideally be mounted in the inspiratory limb of the breathing system

QUESTION 43

A pressure-cycled ventilator

A. Is a minute volume divider
B. Can be cycled from inspiration to expiration after a set time
C. Compensates for small leaks
D. The peak inspiratory pressure is determined by compliance of the patient's lungs
E. A reduced tidal volume will be delivered if the airway resistance increases

QUESTION 44

The paramagnetic principle is used in the following

A. To measure cardiac output
B. In an ultrasonic nebuliser
C. To measure nitric oxide concentration
D. To measure oxygen concentration
E. To measure isoflurane concentration

QUESTION 45

The Severinghaus carbon dioxide electrode

A. Has a surrounding medium of sodium bicarbonate
B. Contains a carbon dioxide sensitive glass
C. Is more accurate with gases than blood
D. Accuracy is affected by nitrous oxide
E. Is temperature sensitive

QUESTION 46

The catheter-transducer system in the direct measurement of arterial pressure should have the following features

A. A stiff diaphragm
B. A short catheter
C. A wide bore catheter
D. A critically damped system (D=1)
E. A continuous slow flow of flush solution through the catheter

QUESTION 47

Concerning the effects of breathing 100% oxygen at normal atmospheric pressure

A. The haemoglobin becomes fully saturated
B. The alveolar PO_2 is approximately 200 mmHg
C. The alveolar PCO_2 is approximately 40 mmHg
D. The oxygen dissolved in the plasma is approximately 20 ml/100ml
E. The total percentage increase of oxygen carried in the blood is about 100%

QUESTION 48

Concerning connections between anaesthetic apparatus

A. All adult facemasks have a 30 mm female opening
B. All adult tracheal tube connectors have a 15 mm male fitting
C. Connectors on scavenging systems have a diameter of 30 mm
D. A size 4 laryngeal mask has a 22 mm diameter connector
E. A size 1 laryngeal mask has a 15 mm diameter connector

QUESTION 49

The ideal oxygen failure warning device

A. Depends on the pressure of a gas other than the oxygen itself
B. Uses a battery rather than mains power
C. Should interrupt the flow of all other gases when activated
D. Gives an audible signal of sufficient duration and volume
E. Should give a warning of impending failure and a further warning that failure has occurred

QUESTION 50

The following are true of a gas cylinder valve

A. The valve should be regularly greased to prevent sticking
B. The valve should be opened quickly to blow off any dirt that may be present in the outlet

C. Should the cylinder valve itself be leaking, it is possible to tighten the packing nut by turning it in a clockwise direction
D. The valve should always be fully open when the cylinder is in use
E. The valve should be left fully open on all empty cylinders

QUESTION 51

In the measurement of a single forced expiration using a spirometer, the following statements are true

A. Normally, the forced expiratory volume in the first second (FEV1) is about 65% of the forced vital capacity (FVC)
B. The FEV1 is reduced much more than the FVC in pulmonary fibrosis
C. Both the FEV1 and FVC are reduced in asthma
D. The FEV1 is directly proportional to the expiratory effort
E. The FVC is often slightly more than the vital capacity measured on a slow exhalation

QUESTION 52

The Bernoulli principle may be utilized in the following

A. Venturi oxygen mask
B. Nebuliser
C. Ventilator
D. TEC 6 vaporiser
E. Humidifier

QUESTION 53

Concerning the Rotameter

A. It consists of a vertical tube with even diameter
B. The pressure drop across the bobbin increases with increasing flow
C. At low flows, the viscosity of the gas becomes important
D. At high flows, the density of the gas becomes important
E. In a hyperbaric chamber, a flowmeter will deliver less gas than the setting indicates

QUESTION 54

The following lung volumes can be measured with a simple spirometer

A. Vital capacity
B. Anatomical dead space
C. Functional residual capacity
D. Residual volume
E. Total lung capacity

QUESTION 55

Pressure can be measured with the following

A. Aneroid gauge
B. Bourdon gauge
C. Rayleigh refractometer
D. Raman gauge
E. Displacement of a flexible diaphragm

QUESTION 56

The Bourdon gauge

A. Consists of a metal bellows
B. Is utilized in anaesthetic ventilators
C. Is suitable for measuring high pressures
D. Can be adapted to measure flow
E. Can be adapted to measure temperature

QUESTION 57

Concerning spectrophotometric absorption spectra of reduced and oxygenated haemoglobin

A. At the isobestic point, the absorption coefficient is the same
B. The isobestic point occurs at a wavelength around 650 nm
C. The amount of oxygenated haemoglobin is directly proportional to the shift in the isobestic point
D. The maximum difference in the absorption of the two forms of haemoglobin occurs at a wavelength around 940 nm
E. The pulse oximeter uses the difference between the absorption spectra of the two forms of Hb to quantify their relative concentrations

QUESTION 58

The following statements are true regarding the capacitor

A. A capacitor consists of two conductor plates separated by an insulator
B. The size of a capacitor depends upon the number of turns of wire wound as a coil
C. The size of a capacitor depends upon the surface area of the plates
D. The size of a capacitor depends upon the thickness of the insulator
E. The unit of capacitance is the joule

QUESTION 59

The following methods can be used to measure the functional residual capacity of the lung

A. Helium dilution
B. Body plethysmograph
C. Nitrogen washout
D. Fowler's method
E. Bohr's method

QUESTION 60

The following are SI base units

A. Ampere
B. Candela
C. Mole
D. Newton
E. Pascal

Exam 3: Answers

QUESTION 1

A. TRUE B. TRUE C. TRUE D. FALSE E. FALSE

If venous access is impossible, the tracheal route may be used for adrenaline, atropine and lignocaine. Drug doses are 2-3 times that of the intravenous route. Drug absorption may be impaired by atelectasis, pulmonary oedema, and in the case of adrenaline, local vasoconstriction. Do not give sodium bicarbonate or calcium chloride/gluconate by this route.

Ref: H G W Paw, G R Park. Drug Prescribing in Anaesthesia and Intensive Care, 1st ed. Greenwich Medical Media, 1996.

QUESTION 2

A. TRUE B. TRUE C. FALSE D. TRUE E. FALSE

Aminophylline is a mixture of theophylline and ethylenediamine, which makes it 20 times more soluble than theophylline alone. Theophylline is a non-specific phosphodiesterase inhibitor. There is debate regarding the mode of action of theophylline in the airways. The increase in intracellular cAMP as a result of phosphodiesterase inhibition is no longer thought to be the mechanism for the bronchodilatation. Other possible mechanisms include adenosine antagonism, calcium blockade and release of catecholamines.

It has a narrow therapeutic index (margin between the therapeutic and toxic dose). Metabolism is decreased in heart failure, cirrhosis, viral infections, and by drugs such as cimetidine, ciprofloxacin, erythromycin, and oral contraceptive (half-life is increased). Metabolism is increased in smokers, heavy drinkers, and by drugs such as phenytoin, carbamazepine, rifampicin, and barbiturates (half-life is decreased). It must be given by slow intravenous injection (over at least 20 minutes) and is too irritant for intramuscular use.

Ref: W McCaughey, R S J Clarke, J P H Fee, W F M Wallace. Anaesthetic Physiology and Pharmacology, 1st ed. Churchill Livingstone, 1997.

QUESTION 3

A. FALSE B. FALSE C. FALSE D. TRUE E. TRUE

Adenosine is effective in SVTs. It depresses the SA node activity and blocks conduction in the AV node, with little effect on conduction through the Purkinje fibres, atria and ventricular tissues. Although it is ineffective in VTs, it can serve to distinguish SVT with associated bundle branch block from VT in a patient with broad complex tachycardia. It has a very short half life

(<10 seconds), and should be given as a rapid i.v. bolus, preferably via a central line. Because of its short half life, any associated side effects (chest discomfort, wheezing and flushing) are brief. It is a potent coronary vasodilator and may cause coronary steal in susceptible patients.

Ref: H G W Paw, G R Park. Drug Prescribing in Anaesthesia and Intensive Care, 1st ed. Greenwich Medical Media, 1996.

QUESTION 4

A. TRUE   B. TRUE   C. TRUE   D. TRUE   E. FALSE

When combined with oxygen it results in the formation of nitrogen dioxide which is toxic. This is a major problem in the use of nitric oxide. When released into the circulation, nitric oxide is rapidly deactivated by haemoglobin.

Ref: R D Miller. Anesthesia, 4th ed. Churchill Livingstone, 1994.

QUESTION 5

A. FALSE   B. FALSE   C. FALSE   D. TRUE   E. FALSE

Dopexamine is a synthetic analogue of dopamine. Dopamine occurs naturally and is a precursor of noradrenaline. Dopexamine exerts ß-2 adrenergic and DA-1 dopaminergic effects, resulting in renal and splanchnic vasodilatation, increased cardiac output, reduced systemic and pulmonary vascular resistance, and reduced atrial filling pressures. It has little ß-1 or α-adrenergic activity.

Ref: H G W Paw, G R Park. Drug Prescribing in Anaesthesia and Intensive Care, 1st ed. Greenwich Medical Media, 1996.

QUESTION 6

A. TRUE   B. FALSE   C. TRUE   D. TRUE   E. FALSE

The interactions between propofol and ketamine, and propofol and alfentanil are additive.

Ref: H R Vinik. Intravenous Anaesthetic Drug Interactions: Practical Applications. European Journal of Anaesthesiology 1995; 12: 13-19.

QUESTION 7

A. TRUE   B. TRUE   C. FALSE   D. FALSE   E. TRUE

Co-proxamol (dextropropoxyphene and paracetamol) is widely available from the pharmacy and is frequently taken in overdose. The initial features are those of acute opioid overdose with respiratory depression, pinpoint pupils and coma. Naloxone is the antidote for dextropropoxyphene. Paracetamol hepatoxicity may develop later and should be treated with either acetylcysteine intravenously or methionine by mouth. Cyanide antidotes include dicobalt edetate, given alone, and sodium nitrite, followed by sodium thiosulphate. Sodium calciumedetate and penicillamine are antidotes for heavy metal poisoning, especially lead. Desferrioxamine is the specific antidote for iron poisoning, which is very common in children. Pralidoxime mesylate, a cholinesterase reactivator, is indicated, as an adjunct to atropine in the treatment of organophosphorus poisoning.

Ref: British National Formulary, 1997

QUESTION 8

A. TRUE B. TRUE C. TRUE D. TRUE E. FALSE

Drugs with substantial first pass metabolism include:-

Aspirin, Codeine, Diltiazem, Glyceryl trinitrate, Hydralazine, Isosorbide dinitrate, Labetalol, Levodopa, Metoprolol, Morphine, Prazosin, Propranolol, Terfenadine, Verapamil.

Ref: W McCaughey, R S J Clarke, J P H Fee, W F M Wallace. Anaesthetic Physiology and Pharmacology, 1st ed. Churchill Livingstone, 1997.

QUESTION 9

A. FALSE B. TRUE C. FALSE D. FALSE E. TRUE

Drugs which increase myocardial contractility are termed positive inotropes. The mechanism of action of positive inotropes can be classified into three groups.

- Increasing intracellular cAMP by activation of adenylcyclase: catecholamines and sympathetic agents.

- Inhibiting phosphodiesterase, the enzyme responsible for breakdown of cAMP: theophylline, amrinone, milrinone and enoximone.

- Increasing intracellular calcium: digoxin.

Ref: W McCaughey, R S J Clarke, J P H Fee, W F M Wallace. Anaesthetic Physiology and Pharmacology, 1st ed. Churchill Livingstone, 1997.

QUESTION 10

A. FALSE B. TRUE C. FALSE D. FALSE E. FALSE

Isoflurane is a halogenated methyl ethyl ether.
The MAC is 1.15% in 100% O_2, decreasing to 0.5% in 70% N_2O.

It is stable in soda–lime, unlike halothane and sevoflurane. It causes slightly more respiratory depression than halothane, although less so than enflurane. Isoflurane and enflurane have the same oil/gas partition coefficient (98).

Ref: A R Aitkenhead, G Smith. Textbook of Anaesthesia, 3rd ed. Churchill Livingstone, 1996.

QUESTION 11

A. FALSE B. TRUE C. TRUE D. TRUE E. TRUE

Hyoscine is more sedative than atropine. Atropine reverses the miosis caused by opioids. The activity of eccrine sweat glands (innervated by cholinergic sympathetic neurones) is inhibited by atropine. In overdose, atropine causes hyperpyrexia via a central effect on temperature-regulating mechanisms but suppression of sweating is a contributing factor. Atropine and hyoscine are both tertiary compounds and readily cross the blood-brain barrier.

Summary of the effects of the three antimuscarinic agents:-

	Atropine	Hyoscine	Glycopyrrolate
Sedation	+	+++	0
Anti-sialagogue	+	+++	++
Increase heart rate	+++	+	++
Relax smooth muscle	++	+	++
Myadriasis	+	+++	0
Prevent motion sickness	+	+++	0

Ref: W McCaughey, R S J Clarke, J P H Fee, W F M Wallace. Anaesthetic Physiology and Pharmacology, 1st ed. Churchill Livingstone, 1997.

QUESTION 12

A. TRUE B. FALSE C. FALSE D. FALSE E. FALSE

MAC is an index of anaesthetic potency and is inversely proportional to lipid solubility (Meyer-Overton theory). It is determined in unpremedicated subjects and does not change with increasing duration of anaesthesia. It is not determined by blood sampling.

Ref: A R Aitkenhead, G Smith. Textbook of Anaesthesia, 3rd ed. Churchill Livingstone, 1996.

QUESTION 13

A. FALSE B. FALSE C. TRUE D. FALSE E. FALSE

Morphine and propranolol have low bioavailability due to substantial hepatic first-pass metabolism. Methadone, in contrast to the other opioids, is well absorbed after oral administration and does not undergo substantial hepatic first-pass metabolism. It therefore has high bioavailability. Atenolol and gentamicin have low bioavailability due to poor absorption after oral administration.

Ref: W McCaughey, R S J Clarke, J P H Fee, W F M Wallace. Anaesthetic Physiology and Pharmacology, 1st ed. Churchill Livingstone, 1997.

QUESTION 14

A. TRUE   B. FALSE   C. FALSE   D. TRUE   E. FALSE

Physostigmine and propranolol are highly lipid–soluble and readily cross the blood–brain barrier. Neostigmine, dopamine and glycopyrollate are highly polar and do not cross the blood–brain barrier readily.

Ref: W McCaughey, R S J Clarke, J P H Fee, W F M Wallace. Anaesthetic Physiology and Pharmacology, 1st ed. Churchill Livingstone, 1997.

QUESTION 15

A. TRUE   B. TRUE   C. FALSE   D. FALSE   E. FALSE

Metabolism of the following drugs are affected by the acetylator status of the individual:-

- Hydralazine
- Isoniazid
- Sulphonamides
- Phenelzine
- Dapsone
- Procainamide

Rapid acetylator status occurs in approximately 40% of the UK population and is inherited in an autosomal dominant pattern. Slow acetylator status occurs in approximately 60% of the UK population and is inherited in an autosomal recessive pattern.

Ref: W McCaughey, R S J Clarke, J P H Fee, W F M Wallace. Anaesthetic Physiology and Pharmacology, 1st ed. Churchill Livingstone, 1997.

QUESTION 16

A. TRUE   B. TRUE   C. FALSE   D. FALSE   E. FALSE

Drugs excreted mostly unchanged by the kidney include:-

Aminoglycoside antibiotics
Cephalosporins
Digoxin
Ephedrine
Lithium
Milrinone
Neostigmine
Penicillins

The significance of these drugs is that they will accumulate in renal impairment.

Ref: W McCaughey, R S J Clarke, J P H Fee, W F M Wallace. Anaesthetic Physiology and Pharmacology, 1st ed. Churchill Livingstone, 1997.

QUESTION 17

A. TRUE   B. TRUE   C. TRUE   D. TRUE   E. TRUE

Amitriptyline is a tricyclic antidepressant. In overdose it causes dry mouth, dilated pupils, urinary retention, hypotension, hypothermia, hyperreflexia, extensor plantar responses, convulsions, respiratory failure, cardiac conduction defects, arrhythmias, metabolic acidosis, and coma of varying degree.

Ref: British National Formulary, 1997

QUESTION 18

A. TRUE   B. TRUE   C. TRUE   D. TRUE   E. TRUE

Ref: W McCaughey, R S J Clarke, J P H Fee, W F M Wallace. Anaesthetic Physiology and Pharmacology, 1st ed. Churchill Livingstone, 1997.

QUESTION 19

A. FALSE   B. TRUE   C. TRUE   D. TRUE   E. FALSE

Verapamil and digoxin are used in supraventricular arrhythmias.

Ref: British National Formulary, 1997

QUESTION 20

A. FALSE   B. FALSE   C. TRUE   D. FALSE   E. TRUE

It is difficult for haemodialysis to remove a drug if its volume of distribution is large. The half-life of a drug is the time taken for the plasma concentration (not clinical effect) to be reduced by half. Administering a drug intravenously gives it 100% bioavailability. Affinity is the ability of the drug to bind to the receptor site. Efficacy is the maximal effect, which a drug is capable of producing, and is represented by the plateau of the dose-response curve. It takes 4-5 half-lives for a drug to achieve steady-state concentration. Therefore, drugs with a long half-life require a loading dose to achieve a more rapid therapeutic concentration.

Ref: W McCaughey, R S J Clarke, J P H Fee, W F M Wallace. Anaesthetic Physiology and Pharmacology, 1st ed. Churchill Livingstone, 1997.

QUESTION 21

A. TRUE   B. FALSE   C. FALSE   D. FALSE   E. TRUE

The bronchioles contribute 10-20% of total airway resistance, the bronchi 30-40%, and the trachea and more proximal structures 50%. The alveoli are lined by 2 types of epithelial cells. Type I pneumocytes are flat cells with large cytoplasmic extensions and are the primary lining cells. Type II pneumocytes, although more numerous than type I cells, cover less of the epithelial lining. These contain numerous lamellar inclusion bodies and are the source of surfactant. The pores of Kohn are holes in the alveolar wall allowing communication between alveoli of adjoining lobules.

Ref: J B West. Respiratory Physiology - the essentials, 5th ed. Williams and Wilkins, 1995.

QUESTION 22

A. TRUE B. TRUE C. TRUE D. FALSE E. TRUE

The neonate has a lower lung compliance but a higher chest wall compliance compared with the adult. Airway resistance is higher as the airways remain relatively narrow. The high airway resistance and low lung compliance result in a short time constant. Ventilation is almost entirely diaphragmatic in comparison with the bucket-handle movement in the adult. Physiological dead space is approximately 30% of the tidal volume as in the adult, but the absolute volume is small, so that any increase caused by apparatus dead space has a disproportionately greater effect on a small child. The respiratory rate is approximately 28 per minute.

Ref: A R Aitkenhead, G Smith. Textbook of Anaesthesia, 3rd ed. Churchill Livingstone, 1996.

QUESTION 23

A. TRUE B. FALSE C. FALSE D. FALSE E. TRUE

Foetal haemoglobin (HbF) forms approximately 80% of haemoglobin at birth. Adult haemoglobin (HbA) haemopoiesis is established fully at 6 months. HbF is made up of two α and two γ chains. HbF has a greater affinity for oxygen than adult haemoglobin (HbA) because it binds less avidly to 2,3-DPG and the dissociation curve is shifted to the left. HbF is present in ß-thalassaemia major and sickle cell anaemia.

Ref: A R Aitkenhead, G Smith. Textbook of Anaesthesia, 3rd ed. Churchill Livingstone, 1996.

QUESTION 24

A. FALSE B. TRUE C. FALSE D. TRUE E. TRUE

ECG changes in hypokalaemia include:-

- Widened QRS complex
- Prolonged QT interval
- ST depression
- Reduced height of T wave
- Increased height of U wave

Ref: A R Aitkenhead, G Smith. Textbook of Anaesthesia, 3rd ed. Churchill Livingstone, 1996.

QUESTION 25

A. FALSE B. FALSE C. TRUE D. TRUE E. TRUE

Lung surfactant is a mixture of lipids and proteins (~10%). Phospholipid, phosphatidyl choline is a major constituent of surfactant. Surfactant is produced by type II pneumocytes in the alveolar epithelium. The major function of surfactant is to reduce surface tension at the air–liquid interface in the alveolus and small airways, thereby improving lung compliance, promoting alveolar stability, and reducing the tendency towards atelectasis at low lung volumes. It may also play a part in keeping the lung tissues dry.

Ref: J B West. Respiratory Physiology - the essentials, 5th ed. Williams and Wilkins, 1995.

QUESTION 26

A. FALSE B. FALSE C. FALSE D. TRUE E. TRUE

Obesity and anaesthesia decreases FRC. FRC remains the same or increases slightly with increasing age. Closing capacity increases to a greater extent than FRC, with increasing age. If closing capacity exceeds FRC (in the supine position after 40 years and in the erect position after 60 years), there will be dependent airway closure during tidal respiration.

Ref: A R Aitkenhead, G Smith. Textbook of Anaesthesia, 3rd ed. Churchill Livingstone, 1996.

QUESTION 27

A. FALSE B. TRUE C. FALSE D. TRUE E. TRUE

The PO_2 of the CSF is lower than that of arterial blood. The pH is lower than arterial blood. There is very little protein in the CSF compared to plasma (300 times less), which makes it a poor buffer. The glucose level in CSF is two-thirds that of blood. The chloride level is higher in the CSF.

Ref: W F Ganong. Review of Medical Physiology, 18th ed. Lange, 1997.

QUESTION 28

A. TRUE B. TRUE C. TRUE D. FALSE E. FALSE

There is no change in HCO_3^- and oxygen saturation with temperature.

QUESTION 29

A. TRUE B. TRUE C. TRUE D. TRUE E. TRUE

The rate of gastric emptying is proportional to the volume of the stomach contents, with approximately 1–3% of the total gastric content reaching the duodenum per minute in an exponential rate. The presence of fat, acid or hypertonic solutions in the duodenum initiates a neurally mediated inhibitory enterogastric reflex, delaying the rate of gastric emptying. Gastric emptying is also under control of the autonomic nervous system. Increased vagal tone hastens gastric emptying. Anti-muscarinic agents therefore delay gastric emptying. Fear, anxiety and pain decrease gastric emptying.

Ref: W F Ganong. Review of Medical Physiology, 18th ed. Lange, 1997.

QUESTION 30

A. FALSE B. TRUE C. FALSE D. FALSE E. FALSE

The total volume of both lungs is the vital capacity plus the residual volume. The volume which may be forcibly exhaled in one second is approximately 75-85% of the vital capacity. The functional residual capacity and residual volume cannot be measured by spirometry. The vital capacity is the sum of the inspiratory reserve volume, expiratory reserve volume and tidal volume.

Ref: J B West. Respiratory Physiology - the essentials, 5th ed. Williams and Wilkins, 1995.

QUESTION 31

A. FALSE B. FALSE C. FALSE D. FALSE E. TRUE

Blood flow through the coronary arteries varies throughout the cycle, about two-thirds occurring in diastole. Normal coronary blood flow at rest is approximately 250 ml/min or 5% of the cardiac output. Hypoxia increases coronary blood flow 2-3 fold. There is a high O_2 extraction rate, therefore, any increase in O_2 demand must be met by increased delivery by way of an increase in coronary blood flow. In aortic stenosis the pressure in the left ventricle must be much higher than that in the aorta to eject the blood. During systole, the coronary vessels are severely compressed resulting in reduced blood flow.

Ref: W F Ganong. Review of Medical Physiology, 18th ed. Lange, 1997.

QUESTION 32

A. TRUE B. FALSE C. TRUE D. TRUE E. FALSE

Alveolar pressure has to be above atmospheric during expiration. Physiological dead space is approximately 30% of tidal volume.

Ref: J B West. Respiratory Physiology - the essentials, 5th ed. Williams and Wilkins, 1995.

QUESTION 33

A. TRUE B. FALSE C. TRUE D. FALSE E. TRUE

The rapid phase of depolarisation is due to an increase in Na^+ permeability. This is followed by a slower increase in Ca^{2+} permeability, which produces the plateau phase. Repolarisation after this plateau is due to a delayed increase in K^+ permeability. The action potential of cardiac muscle differs markedly from skeletal muscle. The duration of depolarisation is approximately 200 ms in contrast to 1-2 ms in skeletal muscle. Cardiac muscle is inexcitable during this period. The refractory period is almost as long as the muscle twitch which it elicits.

Ref: W F Ganong. Review of Medical Physiology, 18th ed. Lange, 1997.

QUESTION 34

A. TRUE B. TRUE C. TRUE D. FALSE E. FALSE

The bundle of His gives off a left bundle branch at the top of the interventricular septum and continues as the right bundle branch. The left bundle branch divides into an anterior fascicle and a posterior fascicle.

Ref: W F Ganong. Review of Medical Physiology, 18th ed. Lange, 1997.

QUESTION 35

A. TRUE B. FALSE C. TRUE D. TRUE E. FALSE

Lipid solubility determines the potency of an inhalational anaesthetic and does not have an influence on the speed of onset of anaesthesia. Increased cardiac output increases the uptake of volatile anaesthetic agents from the alveoli and slows the onset of anaesthesia. This is in contrast to intravenous anaesthetic agents, where increase cardiac output increases the onset of intra-venous anaesthetic agents.

Ref: A R Aitkenhead, G Smith. Textbook of Anaesthesia, 3rd ed. Churchill Livingstone, 1996.

QUESTION 36

A. FALSE B. TRUE C. TRUE D. TRUE E. TRUE

Plasma potassium concentration is a poor reflection of total body potassium. Plasma potassium rises in metabolic acidosis. Potassium enters cells in the presence of insulin. Aldosterone causes sodium retention and potassium loss.

Ref: W F Ganong. Review of Medical Physiology, 18th ed. Lange, 1997.

QUESTION 37

A. TRUE B. FALSE C. TRUE D. TRUE E. FALSE

The calculation of oxygen delivery (DO_2) and oxygen consumption (VO_2) require in addition the cardiac output, mixed venous oxygen saturation and mixed venous oxygen tension.

Ref: A R Aitkenhead, G Smith. Textbook of Anaesthesia, 3rd ed. Churchill Livingstone, 1996.

QUESTION 38

A. FALSE   B. FALSE   C. FALSE   D. FALSE   E. FALSE

The electroencephalogram (EEG) measures the electrical activity in the outermost layers of the grey matter, probably mostly from dendrites. The amplitude of the potential is in the microvolt scale when recorded from the scalp. Alpha waves have an amplitude of approximately 50 microvolts. Alpha rhythm is seen at rest with the mind wandering and eyes closed. The characteristic 3 Hz spike pattern is seen with petit mal. Delta waves are large, slow waves with a frequency of between 0.5-3 Hz.

Ref: W F Ganong. Review of Medical Physiology, 18th ed. Lange, 1997.

QUESTION 39

A. TRUE   B. TRUE   C. FALSE   D. TRUE   E. TRUE

Schwann cells form myelin sheaths around the myelinated neurones. Myelinated neurones are devoid of myelin at the nodes of Ranvier. Nodes of Ranvier are absent in unmyelinated neurones. Unmyelinated neurones still contain Schwann cells, but they do not form a myelin sheath around the axon. The autonomic preganglionic neurones are mostly myelinated B fibres. The postganglionic neurones are mostly unmyelinated C fibres.

Ref: W F Ganong. Review of Medical Physiology, 18th ed. Lange, 1997.

QUESTION 40

A. TRUE   B. TRUE   C. TRUE   D. FALSE   E. FALSE

Sympathetic preganglionic cell bodies lie in the inter-mediolateral columns of the spinal cord between segments T1 to L2 or L3. Parasympathetic outflow come from the mid brain, medulla and spinal segments S2 to S4. Stimulation of the sympathetic innervation of the bronchial smooth muscle causes bronchodilatation. Stimulation of the sympathetic innervation of the stomach causes inhibition of gastric secretion. Some preganglionic sympathetic neurones pass through the paravertebral ganglion chain (without synapsing) and end on postganglionic neurones located in collateral ganglia close to the viscera. Discrete parasympathetic ganglia include ciliary, sphenopalatine, submaxillary and otic ganglia.

Ref: W F Ganong. Review of Medical Physiology, 18th ed. Lange, 1997.

QUESTION 41

A. FALSE   B. TRUE   C. FALSE   D. TRUE   E. TRUE

The function of infrared analysers is based on the fact that gases that have two or more dissimilar atoms in the molecule such as N_2O, CO_2 and all halogenated anaesthetic agents have specific and unique absorption spectra of infrared light. The non-polar molecules of nitrogen, oxygen, helium, argon and xenon do not absorb infrared light and cannot be measured using this technology.

Ref: J A Dorsch, S E Dorsch. Understanding Anaesthesia Equipment: Construction, Care and Complications, 3rd ed. Williams and Wilkins, 1994.

QUESTION 42

A. FALSE B. TRUE C. TRUE D. TRUE E. FALSE

The Wright's respirometer is a vane anemometer. Its function is affected by moisture, which causes the pointer to stick. It should ideally be mounted in the expiratory limb of the breathing system so that leaks which occur in the inspiratory limb are eliminated from the evaluation of expired minute volume.

Ref: J A Dorsch, S E Dorsch. Understanding Anaesthesia Equipment: Construction, Care and Complications, 3rd ed. Williams and Wilkins, 1994.

QUESTION 43

A. FALSE B. FALSE C. TRUE D. FALSE E. TRUE

A pressure-cycled ventilator cycles into expiration when a pre-set airway pressure is achieved. This allows compensation for small leaks. However if the airway resistance increases and/or compliance of the patient deteriorates, a reduced tidal volume will be delivered at the pre-set cycling pressure. In addition, inspiratory time varies with changes in resistance and compliance.

Ref: A R Aitkenhead, G Smith. Textbook of Anaesthesia, 3rd ed. Churchill Livingstone, 1996.

QUESTION 44

A. FALSE B. FALSE C. FALSE D. TRUE E. FALSE

Of the gases of interest in anaesthesia, only oxygen is paramagnetic. Paramagnetic oxygen analysers rely on the magnetic property of the oxygen molecule, whereby it is attracted by a magnetic field. In contrast, most other gases, including nitrous oxide and nitrogen, are weakly diamagnetic and are thus repelled by a magnetic field.

Ref: J A Dorsch, S E Dorsch. Understanding Anaesthesia Equipment: Construction, Care and Complications, 3rd ed. Williams and Wilkins, 1994.

QUESTION 45

A. TRUE B. FALSE C. FALSE D. FALSE E. TRUE

The Severinghaus carbon dioxide electrode provides a direct method of PCO_2 measurement from the $[H^+]$ change. It contains a hydrogen ion sensitive glass, with electrodes either side of it. A thin film of sodium bicarbonate solution surrounds this glass.

Nitrous oxide does not affect the measurement of PCO_2 using the Severinghaus electrode, but will indeed affect the measurement of end-tidal CO_2 using the infrared absorption spectrophotometry.

Ref: P D Davis, G D Parbrook, G N C Kenny. Basic Physics and Measurement in Anaesthesia, 4th ed. Butterworth-Heinemann, 1995.

QUESTION 46

A. TRUE B. TRUE C. TRUE D. FALSE E. TRUE

A recording system must accurately reproduce both the amplitude and phase difference of each harmonic present in the waveform. To achieve this, it is necessary to design a system with a high undamped natural frequency (resonant frequency) and then apply the correct amount of damping. To obtain a high resonant frequency, the diaphragm needs to be stiff and the catheter short and wide. Optimal damping is 64% of critical (D=0.64). This represents the best compromise that can be obtained between the speed of response and the accuracy of registrating the amplitude of the pressure trace. Overdamped systems (due to air bubble or partial blockage of catheter) result in underestimation of systolic pressure and overestimation of diastolic pressure. Underdamped systems (due to low resonant frequency) result in overestimation of systolic pressure and underestimation of diastolic pressure. The mean pressure is not affected by the amount of damping.

An important cause of excess damping is clotting in the arterial cannula. This is minimised by maintaining a slow flow (e.g. 3ml/hr) of flush solution through the catheter using a pressurised reservoir.

Ref: M K Sykes, M D Vickers, C J Hull. Principles of Measurement and Monitoring in Anaesthesia and Intensive Care, 3rd ed. Blackwell, 1991.

QUESTION 47

A. TRUE B. FALSE C. TRUE D. FALSE E. FALSE

The amount of oxygen dissolved in the plasma is 0.3 ml/100ml, and the total oxygen content (dissolved plus combined) is 20 ml/100 ml of blood. Breathing pure oxygen, the partial pressure of oxygen in the alveoli rises from 100 to 673 mmHg, an increase of 6.7 times. As a result, the dissolved oxygen rises to 2 ml/100 ml. The haemoglobin becomes fully saturated and the additional amount of oxygen now carried in the blood as a result of breathing pure oxygen is 2.5 ml/100 ml of blood. The total percentage increase of oxygen carried in the blood is only about 10%. There is no significant change in the alveolar PCO_2 (approximately 40 mmHg) from breathing air.

Ref: D W Hill. Physics Applied to Anaesthesia, 4th ed. Butterworths, 1980.

QUESTION 48

A. FALSE B. TRUE C. TRUE D. FALSE E. TRUE

All adult facemasks have a 22 mm female opening.
All adult tracheal tube connectors have a 15 mm male fitting.
Connectors on scavenging systems have a diameter of 30 mm to ensure that inappropriate connections with anaesthetic apparatus cannot be made.
All laryngeal masks have a 15 mm diameter male connector.

Ref: A R Aitkenhead, G Smith. Textbook of Anaesthesia, 3rd ed. Churchill Livingstone, 1996.

QUESTION 49

A. FALSE B. FALSE C. TRUE D. TRUE E. TRUE

The ideal oxygen failure warning device does not depend on the pressure of any gas other than the oxygen itself, and does not use a battery or mains power.

Ref: A R Aitkenhead, G Smith. Textbook of Anaesthesia, 3rd ed. Churchill Livingstone, 1996.

QUESTION 50

A. FALSE B. FALSE C. TRUE D. TRUE E. FALSE

Valves, regulators, gauges and fittings should never be permitted to come into contact with oils, greases, organic lubricants, rubber or any other combustible substance. A cylinder valve should always be opened slowly. If gas passes quickly into the space between the valve and the yoke or regulator, the rapid recompression in this space will generate large amounts of heat. Because there is little time for dissipation of this heat, this constitutes an adiabatic process (one in which heat is neither lost nor gained from the surroundings). Particles of dust or grease present in this space may be ignited by the heat, causing a fire or an explosion. The valve should always be fully open when the cylinder is in use. Marginal opening may result in failure to deliver adequate gas. Valves should be completely closed on all empty cylinders. Often, cylinders are not completely empty and accidents have resulted from release of gas from a supposedly empty cylinder. If the valve is left open on an empty cylinder, debris and contaminants could be sucked into it when the temperature changes.

Ref: J A Dorsch, S E Dorsch. Understanding Anaesthesia Equipment: Construction, Care and Complications, 3rd ed. Williams and Wilkins, 1994

QUESTION 51

A. FALSE B. FALSE C. TRUE D. FALSE E. FALSE

A very useful and simple test of pulmonary function is the measurement of a single forced expiration. Normally, the forced expiratory volume in the first second (FEV1) is about 75-80% of the forced vital capacity (FVC).

In restrictive diseases such as pulmonary fibrosis both FEV1 and FVC are reduced, but the FEV1/FVC ratio is normal or increased. In obstructive diseases such as asthma and emphysema, the FEV1 is reduced much more than the FVC, giving a low FEV1/FVC ratio.

The FEV1 is reduced by an increase in airway resistance (asthma) or a reduction in elastic recoil of the lung (emphysema). It is remarkably independent of expiratory effort. The FVC is often slightly less than the vital capacity measured on a slow exhalation.

QUESTION 52

A. TRUE   B. TRUE   C. TRUE   D. FALSE   E. TRUE

Ref: A R Aitkenhead, G Smith. Textbook of Anaesthesia, 3rd ed. Churchill Livingstone, 1996.

QUESTION 53

A. FALSE   B. FALSE   C. TRUE   D. TRUE   E. TRUE

The Rotameter consists of a vertical tapered tube that has its smallest diameter at the bottom. The bobbin floats freely in the tube at an equilibrium position where the downward force on it caused by gravity is equal to the upward force caused by gas molecules hitting the bottom of the bobbin. In the variable orifice flowmeter, the annular cross-sectional area varies while the pressure drop across the bobbin remains constant for all positions in the tube. With a longer and narrower constriction (at low flow), flow is a function of the viscosity of the gas (Poiseuille's law). When the constriction is shorter and wider (at high flow), flow depends on the density of the gas (Graham's law).

Flowmeters are calibrated at atmospheric pressure. Pressure changes will affect both the viscosity and the density of a gas and so influence the accuracy of the indicated flow rate. In a hyperbaric chamber, a flowmeter will deliver less gas than the setting indicates. With decreasing barometric pressure (as happens with increasing altitude), the actual flow rate will be higher than the flowmeter reading.

Ref: J A Dorsch, S E Dorsch. Understanding Anaesthesia Equipment: Construction, Care and Complications, 3rd ed. Williams and Wilkins, 1994.

QUESTION 54

A. TRUE   B. FALSE   C. FALSE   D. FALSE   E. FALSE

The volume of the anatomical dead space can be measured by Fowler's method. Neither the functional residual capacity nor the residual volume can be measured with a simple spirometer. Since the total lung capacity is the sum of the residual volume, it too cannot be obtained using a simple spirometer.

Ref: J B West. Respiratory Physiology - the essentials, 5th ed. Williams and Wilkins, 1995.

QUESTION   55

A. TRUE   B. TRUE   C. FALSE   D. FALSE   E. TRUE

High pressures commonly employed in anaesthetic practice can be measured using a Bourdon gauge. In this gauge, the gas at high pressure causes a tube to uncoil and in doing so moves a pointer over a scale on a dial. Bourdon gauges have the advantage over manometers that there is no liquid to spill, and they are sometimes called anaeroid gauges from the Greek 'a-neros' (without liquid). Another form of anaeroid gauge is based on a bellows or capsule which expands or contracts depending on the pressure across it. The strain gauge pressure transducer involves movement of a diaphragm with changes in pressure. This movement of the diaphragm alters the tension in the resistance wire thus changing its resistance. The change of current flow through the resistor can then be amplified and displayed as a measure of pressure on a scale. The Rayleigh refractometer and Raman spectrophotometer are techniques used for anaesthetic gas analysis.

Ref: P D Davis, G D Parbrook, G N C Kenny. Basic Physics and Measurement in Anaesthesia, 4th ed. Butterworth-Heinemann, 1995.

QUESTION   56

A. FALSE   B. FALSE   C. TRUE   D. TRUE   E. TRUE

The Bourdon gauge consists of a coiled tube which is flattened in cross-section. One end of the coil is anchored to the case and connected to the source of pressure, whilst the other end is closed and attached to a mechanism which drives the pointer across a dial.

Pressure gauges on anaesthetic ventilators usually comprise a simple bellows of aneroid gauge whilst high gas pressures (e.g. in medical cylinders) are measured using the Bourdon gauge. It can also be adapted for measuring flow and temperature. The Bourdon gauge flowmeter is used to sense the pressure drop across an orifice. In the Bourdon gauge thermometer, the change in pressure produced by the alteration in temperature is sensed by the gauge and displayed on the dial. This type of thermometer is robust but not very accurate. It is generally employed to measure fairly large temperature changes, e.g. in autoclaves.

Ref: M K Sykes, M D Vickers, C J Hull. Principles of Measurement and Monitoring in Anaesthesia and Intensive Care, 3rd ed. Blackwell, 1991.

QUESTION   57

A. TRUE   B. FALSE   C. FALSE   D. TRUE   E. TRUE

At the isobestic point, the absorption coefficients are identical. This occurs at a wavelength of 800 nm.

The maximum difference in the absorption of the two forms of haemoglobin occurs at a wavelength of about 650 nm. The pulse oximeter probe contains two light-emitting diodes, one for red (660 nm) and one for infrared (940 nm) light. This technique utilizes the difference between the characteristic absorption spectra of the two forms of haemoglobin to quantify their relative concentrations

Ref: M K Sykes, M D Vickers, C J Hull. Principles of Measurement and Monitoring in Anaesthesia and Intensive Care, 3rd ed. Blackwell, 1991.

QUESTION 58

A. TRUE B. FALSE C. TRUE D. TRUE E. FALSE

A capacitor consists of two conductors separated by an insulator, known as the dielectric. In its simplest form, this consists of two metal plates separated by a thin layer of air. The size of a capacitor determines the quantity of electricity it can store for a given charge potential, and depends upon the surface area of the plates, the thickness of the insulator, and its ability to store charge. The unit of capacitance is the Farad (F).

Ref: M K Sykes, M D Vickers, C J Hull. Principles of Measurement and Monitoring in Anaesthesia and Intensive Care, 3rd ed. Blackwell, 1991.

QUESTION 59

A. TRUE B. TRUE C. TRUE D. FALSE E. FALSE

Fowler's method is used to measure the anatomical dead space, whilst Bohr's method is used to measure physiological dead space. Although Fowler's method is also an analysis of nitrogen washout, the method of measurement of functional residual capacity is different. To obtain the FRC, 100% oxygen is inspired at the end of a normal expiration (at FRC). The total volume of expired gas over several minutes is then analysed for its nitrogen content. Since this amount of nitrogen was originally contained in the FRC to give a nitrogen concentration of 79%, the FRC can be derived.

The two other methods for measuring FRC involve the use of helium dilution and the body plethysmograph.

Ref: J B West. Respiratory Physiology - the essentials, 5th ed. Williams and Wilkins, 1995.

QUESTION 60

A. TRUE B. TRUE C. TRUE D. FALSE E. FALSE

There are seven base units (ampere, candela, Kelvin, kilogram, metre, mole and second) from which several other units are derived. The unit of force is the newton (N). This is the force required to accelerate a mass of 1 kg at a rate of 1 metre per second and is expressed in terms of $m.kg.s^{-2}$. The unit of pressure, the Pascal (Pa), can be represented in base units as $m^{-1}.kg.s^{-2}$.

Ref: M K Sykes, M D Vickers, C J Hull. Principles of Measurement and Monitoring in Anaesthesia and Intensive Care, 3rd ed. Blackwell, 1991.

Exam 4

QUESTION 1

Regarding rocuronium

A. It is an aminosteroid
B. At a dose of ED95, intubation can be achieved in 60 seconds
C. The main mode of its metabolism is ester hydrolysis
D. The metabolite has significant muscle relaxant activity
E. It is a trigger agent for malignant hyperthermia

QUESTION 2

Drugs with greater than 50% protein binding include

A. Bupivacaine
B. Alfentanil
C. Fentanyl
D. Morphine
E. Warfarin

QUESTION 3

The following local anaesthetic agents are esters

A. Amethocaine
B. Chloroprocaine
C. Cocaine
D. Ropivacaine
E. Prilocaine

QUESTION 4

Drugs capable of producing extrapyramidal side-effects include

A. Amitriptyline
B. Prochlorperazine
C. Droperidol
D. Haloperidol
E. Cyclizine

QUESTION 5

The following drugs decrease intraocular pressure

A. Enflurane
B. Nitrous oxide
C. Etomidate
D. Ketamine
E. Suxamethonium

QUESTION 6

The following drugs increase intracranial pressure

A. Thiopentone
B. Enflurane
C. Propofol
D. Nitrous oxide
E. Pancuronium

QUESTION 7

Regarding log dose-response curves

A. Potency is the ability of a drug to produce maximal response
B. A partial agonist binds to the receptor with a lower affinity than an agonist
C. In the presence of a competitive antagonist the log dose-response curve for an agonist shows a parallel shift to the right
D. In the presence of a non-competitive antagonist, the log dose-response curve for an agonist is shifted to the left
E. A partial agonist can act as a competitive antagonist to a full agonist

QUESTION 8

Drugs contraindicated in malignant hyperthermia include

A. Droperidol
B. Ketamine
C. Etomidate
D. Atropine
E. Lignocaine

QUESTION 9

Drugs contraindicated in porphyria include

A. Lignocaine
B. Etomidate
C. Diclofenac
D. Co-proxamol
E. Propofol

QUESTION 10

In the Vaughan-Williams classification of anti-arrhythmic drugs

A. Digoxin is a class III drug
B. Adenosine is a class Ia drug
C. Flecainide is a class IV drug
D. Lignocaine is a class Ib drug
E. Amiodarone is a class III drug

QUESTION 11

Drugs which may increase serum potassium concentration include

A. Suxamethonium
B. Lisinopril
C. Nifedipine
D. Digoxin
E. Bumetanide

QUESTION 12

Nitrous oxide

A. Is manufactured by fractional distillation of air
B. Is approximately 20 times as soluble as nitrogen in the blood
C. Has a greater density than air
D. Has a direct myocardial depressant effect
E. Sensitizes the myocardium to catecholamines

QUESTION 13

The following are anti-hypertensive agents

A. Moxonidine
B. Pentolamine
C. Phenoxybenzamine
D. Prazosin
E. Losartan

QUESTION 14

The following drugs may increase plasma urea concentration in the presence of normal renal function

A. Tetracycline
B. Frusemide
C. Corticosteroid
D. Captopril
E. Spironolactone

QUESTION 15

The following interactions are antagonistic

A. Nalaxone and dextropropoxyphe.
B. Acetylcysteine and paracetamol
C. Atenolol and salbutamol
D. Protamine and warfarin
E. Tranexamic acid and streptokinase

QUESTION 16

The following non-depolarising muscle relaxants are aminosteroids

A. Pancuronium
B. Atracurium
C. Vecuronium
D. Mivacurium
E. Rocuronium

QUESTION 17

Frusemide

A. Has a duration of 24 hours when given orally
B. Should be given in lower doses in renal impairment
C. May cause hyperuricaemia
D. May cause hypomagnesaemia
E. May cause hypochloraemic alkalosis

QUESTION 18

Dantrolene

A. Can be administered intramuscularly
B. Contains 3 g mannitol in each 20 mg vial of Dantrium
C. The dose for the treatment of malignant hyperthermia should not exceed 1mg/kg in 24 hours
D. Interacts with verapamil
E. Causes hyperkalaemia

QUESTION 19

The action of non-depolarising muscle relaxant is prolonged by

A. Hyponatraemia
B. Hyperkalaemia
C. Hypermagnesaemia
D. Lithium
E. Gentamicin

QUESTION 20

The following drugs have a volume of distribution greater than 100 litres in a 70 kg adult

A. Atracurium
B. Vecuronium
C. Digoxin
D. Thiopentone
E. Fentanyl

QUESTION 21

The following delay the rate of gastric emptying

A. Pain
B. Hypertonic solution
C. Anxiety
D. Hyoscine
E. Fatty food

QUESTION 22

The following intravenous fluids have an acidic pH

A. Haemaccel
B. 0.9% saline
C. 5% glucose in water
D. 4% glucose in 0.18% saline
E. Hartmann's (compound sodium lactate)

QUESTION 23

The following are typical in the elderly patient

A. Body water increases
B. Closing capacity increases
C. Functional residual capacity decreases
D. Glomerular filtration rate remains normal
E. Systolic blood pressure is greater than that of a 30 year old

QUESTION 24

Effects of positive end-expiratory pressure (PEEP) include

A. Increased airway pressure
B. Reduction of cardiac output
C. Increase in cerebral venous pressure
D. Decrease in end tidal CO_2
E. Decreased antidiuretic hormone secretion

QUESTION 25

The following are excitatory transmitters in the CNS

A. Glycine
B. Aspartate
C. Glutamate
D. γ-aminobutyric acid (GABA)
E. 5-Hydroxytryptamine (5-HT)

QUESTION 26

Storage of blood for transfusion causes

A. Raised pH
B. Raised PCO_2
C. Raised plasma bicarbonate
D. Raised plasma dextrose
E. Raised 2,3-Diphosphoglycerate

QUESTION 27

The following may be used to identify cerebrospinal fluid (CSF) after a suspected dural tap

A. CSF forms a cloudy precipitate when mixed with bupivacaine
B. CSF turns thiopentone pink
C. CSF turns litmus paper pink
D. CSF forms a cloudy precipitate with suxamethonium
E. CSF is straw coloured

QUESTION 28

The following statements are true

A. Renin is released by the juxta-glomerular cells
B. Angiotensinogen is made in the liver
C. Angiotensin I is converted in the lungs to Angiotensin II
D. Antagonism of Angiotensin II results in hypotension
E. Aldosterone is produced from zona glomerulosa of the adrenal cortex

QUESTION 29

Vasopressin (ADH)

A. Secretion is decreased by hypovolaemia
B. Secretion is increased in response to an increased in plasma osmolality
C. Is secreted at a constant rate throughout the day and night
D. Increases the permeability of the collecting ducts to water
E. Acts by increasing the formation of cyclic-AMP in the collecting duct cells

QUESTION 30

Insulin

A. Is antagonised by growth hormone
B. Facilitates protein anabolism
C. Promotes glycogen synthesis in the liver
D. Facilitates the deposition of fat
E. Inhibits the passage of potassium ions into cells

QUESTION 31

The following are produced by the adrenal medulla

A. Noradrenaline
B. Dehydroepiandrosterone
C. Prolactin
D. Angiotensin II
E. Deoxycorticosterone

QUESTION 32

Pulmonary surfactant

A. Reduces surface tension at the air-liquid interface in the alveolus
B. Increases lung compliance
C. Promotes alveolar stability
D. Humidifies inspired air
E. Removes inhaled particles under 2 μm in diameter

QUESTION 33

Disorders in which there is an abnormal amino acid substitution in the haemoglobin chain include

A. Methaemoglobinaemia
B. Sickle-cell trait
C. β-thalassaemia
D. Hereditory spherocytosis
E. Glucose-6-phophate dehydrogenase deficiency

QUESTION 34

The following may cause an elevated blood urea

A. Dehydration
B. Infection
C. Steroid therapy
D. Tetracycline therapy
E. Renal disease

QUESTION 35

The following conditions may produce a raised serum alkaline phosphatase

A. Obstructive jaundice
B. Paget's disease
C. Osteoporosis
D. Adolescence
E. Pregnancy

QUESTION 36

In the first 24 hours of fasting

A. Hypoglycaemia occurs
B. The hepatic glycogen store is adequate
C. Gluconeogenesis occurs
D. Lipogenesis occurs
E. Central nervous metabolism changes from ketone bodies to glucose

QUESTION 37

Nutrition in a 70 kg man

A. Fat is an efficient way of storing energy
B. Carbohydrate stores are the major source of fuel
C. Average daily energy intake is 1000 kcal
D. Daily protein requirement is 40 g
E. Linoleic acid is an essential fatty acid

QUESTION 38

The following are reasons why oxygen desaturation is more rapid in a pregnant woman than a non-pregnant woman during apnoea

A. Decreased functional residual capacity
B. Increased oxygen consumption
C. Oxyhaemoglobin dissociation curve is shifted to the right
D. Decreased tidal volume
E. Decreased airway resistance

QUESTION 39

The neonate

A. Has a lower chest wall compliance than that of an adult
B. Has a lower lung compliance than that of an adult
C. Usually increases its cardiac output by increasing heart rate and not stroke volume
D. Has a higher metabolic rate than an adult
E. Has a blood volume of approximately 70 ml/kg

QUESTION 40

ECG changes with hyperkalaemia include

A. A tented T wave
B. A prolonged PR interval
C. A reduced P wave
D. A widened QRS complex
E. A sine wave pattern

QUESTION 41

The following parameters are required for the measurement of oxygen consumption

A. Cardiac index
B. Haemoglobin concentration
C. PaO_2
D. PvO_2
E. Basal metabolic rate

QUESTION 42

Pulmonary capillary wedge pressure does not reflect left ventricular end-diastolic pressure in the following conditions

A. When the catheter tip is positioned in West's zone III
B. Mitral stenosis
C. Aortic regurgitation
D. Pneumonectomy
E. Pulmonary embolus

QUESTION 43

Causes of inaccuracy in thermodilution cardiac output measurements

A. Tricuspid regurgitation
B. Atrial septal defect
C. Ventricular septal defect
D. Atrial fibrillation
E. Fluid being injected through side-port of a percutaneous sheath

QUESTION 44

Isoflurane can be measured using

A. A paramagnetic gas analyser
B. An ultraviolet gas analyser
C. A Raman spectrometer
D. Photoacoustic spectroscopy
E. Mass spectrometry

QUESTION 45

Concerning the measurement of oxygen using the paramagnetic technique

A. The glass spheres are filled with oxygen
B. This technique utilizes the unique property of oxygen to be strongly attracted to a magnetic field
C. The displacing force exerted by the oxygen molecules is related to the concentration of oxygen
D. Inaccuracy occurs in the presence of nitrous oxide
E. Inaccuracy occurs in the presence of water vapour

QUESTION 46

The following conditions result in a high pulmonary capillary wedge pressure

A. Adult respiratory distress syndrome
B. Left ventricular failure
C. Pulmonary hypertension
D. Pulmonary embolus
E. Tricuspid regurgitation

QUESTION 47

Concerning the anaesthetic machine

A. The non–return pressure relief valve is situated upstream of the vaporisers
B. The function of the non–return pressure relief valve is to protect the patient from barotrauma
C. When the emergency oxygen flush is activated, flow bypasses the flowmeters and the vaporisers
D. The use of the emergency oxygen flush leads to dilution of the anaesthetic gases
E. On the flowmeter panel, oxygen is the last gas to be added to the mixture delivered to the back bar

QUESTION   48

Concerning medical gas cylinders

A. Cylinders are made of titanium/aluminium alloy
B. The colour and shape of the plastic disc around the neck of the cylinder identifies the gas it contains
C. Cylinders attached to the anaesthetic machine are usually size E
D. The filling ratio is the weight of the fluid in the cylinder divided by the weight of the cylinder and fluid together
E. Tare weight is the weight of the cylinder when full

QUESTION   49

Regarding the Desflurane Tec 6 vaporiser

A. The vaporiser requires a special adapter to allow mounting onto the Selectatec system
B. The vaporisation chamber is heated to a temperature of 25°C.
C. The vaporisation chamber is pressurised to approximately 2 bar
D. The percentage control dial calibration ranges from 0-8%
E. The fresh gas flow does not enter the vaporisation chamber

QUESTION   50

Regarding the Cardiff Aldasorber

A. It contains activated zeolite
B. It absorbs nitrous oxide with reasonable efficiency
C. It changes colour when exhausted
D. It does not remove carbon dioxide
E. Heating the canister causes the release of the absorbed agents

QUESTION   51

Regarding arterial blood gas measurement

A. Excess heparin lowers the pH of the sample
B. The presence of air bubbles in the sample decreases the oxygen partial pressure
C. The presence of air bubbles in the sample decreases the carbon dioxide partial pressure
D. An old blood sample has a lower pH
E. Base excess is a derived measurement

QUESTION 52

A volatile liquid is allowed to equilibrate with a mixture of gases. The resultant partial pressure of the vapour will depend on

A. The ambient pressure
B. The ambient temperature
C. The surface area of the liquid
D. The volume of the liquid
E. The composition of the different gases.

QUESTION 53

Concerning the measurement of expired carbon dioxide using the infrared absorption technique

A. The wavelength of infrared light used is 4,300 nm
B. The absorption of infrared light by carbon dioxide is based on the Beer–Lambert law
C. The windows on the sample chamber are made of lead crystal glass
D. Nitrous oxide interferes with infrared absorption by carbon dioxide
E. Oxygen interferes with infrared absorption by carbon dioxide

QUESTION 54

The following can be used to measure carbon dioxide in expired gases (capnography)

A. Clark polarographic electrode
B. Paramagnetic analyser
C. Infrared absorption spectrometry
D. Mass spectrometry
E. Raman analyser

QUESTION 55

Concerning the ECG

A. The P wave represents atrial depolarisation
B. The PR interval starts from the beginning of the P wave and ends at the end of the R deflection
C. A QRS complex greater than 0.12 seconds represents conduction delay
D. The T wave represents ventricular depolarisation
E. A normal ECG may be present when the circulation is grossly inadequate

QUESTION 56

Concerning the Clark PO₂ electrode

A. It is an electric cell composed of a platinum cathode and a gold anode
B. An oxygen consuming electrochemical reaction takes place at the anode
C. It can be used to measure oxygen partial pressure in gases and liquids
D. It requires a voltage of 0.6 V to be applied between its electrodes
E. It is sensitive to changes in temperature

QUESTION 57

Electrical diathermy

A. Has a current frequency of 50-60 Hz
B. Has a lower frequency when used for coagulation than when used for cutting
C. In the monopolar type, has a low current density in the active electrode
D. In the monopolar type, is likely to raise the impedance of the circuit as a result of poor plate contact
E. May cause a burn to the tracheal mucosa if the tracheal tube is earthed via the anaesthetic machine

QUESTION 58

Regarding defibrillation of the heart

A. A capacitor is an important component of a defibrillator
B. The amount of current flowing through the heart depends on the energy of the shock and transthoracic impedance
C. Electrode pad size is an important determinant of transthoracic current flow
D. The optimum duration of the output waveform is between 4 and 12 ms
E. The output waveform of most conventional external defibrillators is biphasic

QUESTION 59

The pressure gauge on a nitrous oxide cylinder reads 50 bar. It may be

A. Full
B. Three quarters full
C. Half full
D. One quarter full
E. Supplying a flow of 10 l/min for 30 min

QUESTION   60

The following are true regarding the measurement of compliance of the lungs and chest wall

A. Compliance is the change in airway pressure per unit change in lung volume
B. Compliance is a static measure of lung and chest recoil
C. A patient with only one lung has a compliance of approximately half that of a patient with both lungs
D. Compliance is slightly greater when measured during deflation than when measured during inflation
E. Compliance is decreased in emphysema

Exam 4: Answers

QUESTION 1

A. TRUE   B. FALSE   C. FALSE   D. FALSE   E. FALSE

Rocuronium is an aminosteroid. The ED95 for rocuronium is 0.3 mg/kg. 2 × ED95 (0.6 mg/kg) is required to give a mean onset time of 75 sec. 4 × ED95 gives a mean onset time of 60 sec which is similar to that of suxamethonium. Rocuronium has a hydroxyl group at the 3-carbon position; unlike vecuronium, it will not undergo de-acetylation to produce a 3-OH metabolite with neuromuscular blocking activity.

Ref: J M Hunter. Rocuronium: the newest aminosteroid neuromuscular blocking drug. British Journal of Anaesthesia 1996; 76: 481-483.

QUESTION 2

A. TRUE   B. TRUE   C. TRUE   D. FALSE   E. TRUE

Drug	% protein binding
Warfarin	99
Diazepam	98
Bupivacaine	95
Alfentanil	91
Propofol	90
Fentanyl	85
Thiopentone	80
Lignocaine	65
Morphine	40

Ref: W McCaughey, R S J Clarke, J P H Fee, W F M Wallace. Anaesthetic Physiology and Pharmacology, 1st ed. Churchill Livingstone, 1997.

QUESTION 3

A. TRUE   B. TRUE   C. TRUE   D. FALSE   E. FALSE

Amides	Esters
Bupivacaine	Amethocaine
Lignocaine	Benzocaine
Mepivacaine	Cocaine
Prilocaine	Chloroprocaine
Ropivacaine	Procaine

Classification of local anaesthetics into esters or amides depends on the structure of interme-diate chain in the link. Amides are principally metabolised in the liver and systemic toxicity is more common. Esters are rapidly metabolised and systemic toxicity is rare. Problems with esters include allergic reactions and lack of stability.

Ref: A R Aitkenhead, G Smith. Textbook of Anaesthesia, 3rd ed. Churchill Livingstone, 1996.

QUESTION 4

A. FALSE B. TRUE C. TRUE D. TRUE E. FALSE

Extrapyramidal side-effect is a consequence of the mode of action of drugs which act by inter-fering with dopaminergic transmission in the brain by blocking dopamine receptors. They are caused by the phenothiazines (chlorpromazine, fluphenazine, perphenazine, perchlorperazine and trifluoperazine) and the butyrophenones (droperidol, haloperidol, trifluperidol). Amitriptyline is a tricyclic anti-depressant which does not cause extrapyramidal side-effects, but more commonly produces antimuscarinic side-effects (drowsiness, dry mouth, blurred vision, constipation and urinary retention). Cyclizine is an antihistamine and does not cause extrapyramidal side effects.

Ref: British National Formulary, 1997

QUESTION 5

A. TRUE B. FALSE C. TRUE D. FALSE E. FALSE

Changes in intraocular pressure:

Decrease	Increase	No change
Halothane	Suxamethonium	Nitrous oxide
Enflurane	Ketamine	Atracurium
Isoflurane		Vecuronium
Propofol		
Etomidate		
Thiopentone		

Ref: A R Aitkenhead, G Smith. Textbook of Anaesthesia, 3rd ed. Churchill Livingstone, 1996.

QUESTION 6

A. FALSE B. TRUE C. FALSE D. TRUE E. FALSE

Changes in intracranial pressure:

Decrease	Increase	No change
Propofol	Halothane	Atracurium
Etomidate	Enflurane	Vecuronium

Thiopentone	Isoflurane	Pancuronium
	Nitrous oxide	
	Ketamine	

Ref: A R Aitkenhead, G Smith. Textbook of Anaesthesia, 3rd ed. Churchill Livingstone, 1996.

QUESTION 7

A. FALSE B. FALSE C. TRUE D. FALSE E. TRUE

Potency is the dose (mg/kg) required to produce a given effect. Morphine and fentanyl have similar efficacy, but fentanyl is approximately 100 times more potent than morphine (10 mg of morphine is equivalent to 0.1 mg of fentanyl). Efficacy or intrinsic activity is the ability of a drug to produce maximal response. Agonists are drugs that produce the maximal response. Partial agonists cannot produce a maximal response, though they may bind to the receptor with the same affinity as agonists. In the presence of a competitive antagonist the log dose-response curve shows a parallel shift to the right so that a higher concentration of agonist is required to achieve the same response. In the presence of a non-competitive antagonist the log dose-response curve is shifted to the right and the maximal response is reduced. A partial agonist, by binding to receptors but failing to produce a maximal response, can act as a competitive antagonist to a full agonist.

Ref: W McCaughey, R S J Clarke, J P H Fee, W F M Wallace. Anaesthetic Physiology and Pharmacology, 1st ed. Churchill Livingstone, 1997.

QUESTION 8

A. FALSE B. FALSE C. FALSE D. FALSE E. FALSE

Known triggering agents:-
All inhalational anaesthetic agents
Suxamethonium

Drugs known to be safe:-
Atropine, Benzodiazepines, Bupivacaine, Droperidol, Etomidate, Ketamine, Lignocaine, Nitrous oxide, Non-depolarising muscle relaxant, Opioids, Propofol, Thiopentone

QUESTION 9

A. TRUE B. TRUE C. TRUE D. TRUE E. FALSE

Drugs unsafe in acute porphyrias:-
Amiodarone, Barbiturates, Benzodiazepines, Clonidine, Cocaine, Dextropropoxyphene (Co-proxamol), Diclofenac, Etomidate, Lignocaine, Prilocaine, Ranitidine

Bupivacaine is thought to be safe.

Status epilepticus has been treated successfully with i.v. diazepam. Temazepam is thought to be safe.

Ref: British National Formulary, 1997

QUESTION 10

A. FALSE   B. FALSE   C. FALSE   D. TRUE   E. TRUE

Vaughan-Williams classification of anti-arrhythmic drugs:

Class I	Membrane-stabilising drugs
	Ia: Quinidine, disopyramide, procainamide
	Ib: Lignocaine, mexiletine
	Ic: Flecainide
Class II	ß-blockers
Class III	Amiodarone, bretylium, sotalol (also Class II)
Class IV	Calcium-channel blockers

Digoxin and adenosine are not included in the Vaughan-Williams classification.

Ref: W McCaughey, R S J Clarke, J P H Fee, W F M Wallace. Anaesthetic Physiology and Pharmacology, 1st ed. Churchill Livingstone, 1997.

QUESTION 11

A. TRUE   B. TRUE   C. FALSE   D. FALSE   E. FALSE

Suxamethonium usually results in an increase in serum potassium of approximately 0.5 mmol/l. Lisinopril (ACE inhibitor) may result in hyperkalaemia especially in renal impairment. Frusemide and bumetanide are loop diuretics, which may cause hypokalaemia, hyponatraemia, hypomagnesaemia, hypochloraemic alkalosis and increased calcium excretion.

Potassium-sparing diuretics include amiloride, triamterene, spironolactone, and potassium canrenoate.

Ref: British National Formulary, 1997

QUESTION 12

A. FALSE   B. FALSE   C. TRUE   D. TRUE   E. FALSE

Nitrous oxide is prepared commercially by heating ammonium nitrate. It is approximately 34 times as soluble as nitrogen in the blood, and so diffuses into any air-containing cavity more rapidly, in proportion to its partial pressure in the blood, than nitrogen will exit. The specific gravity of nitrous oxide is 1.53 (air=1). The greater density of nitrous oxide produces slightly more airway resistance than oxygen or air. Nitrous oxide has a direct myocardial depressant effect and a sympathomimetic effect. It does not sensitise the myocardium to catecholamines.

Ref: W McCaughey, R S J Clarke, J P H Fee, W F M Wallace. Anaesthetic Physiology and Pharmacology, 1st ed. Churchill Livingstone, 1997.

QUESTION 13

A. TRUE B. TRUE C. TRUE D. TRUE E. TRUE

Moxonidine, a centrally acting drug has been introduced recently for mild to moderate essential hypertension. Pentolamine is a short-acting α-blocker used to treat hypertensive episodes during surgery for phaeochromocytoma. It is rarely used as a suppression test for the diagnosis of phaeochromocytoma. Phenoxybenzamine is a powerful β-blocker with many side-effects. Its use is usually restricted to the preoperative management of phaeochromocytoma. Prazosin is a post-synaptic α-blocker which rarely causes reflex tachycardia. Losartan is a specific angiotensin-II receptor antagonist with properties similar to those of the ACE inhibitors. However, unlike ACE inhibitors, it does not inhibit the breakdown of bradykinin and other kinins, and thus does not appear to cause a persistent dry cough.

Ref: British National Formulary, 1997

QUESTION 14

A. TRUE B. FALSE C. TRUE D. FALSE E. FALSE

Tetracyclines and steroids may increase plasma urea concentration due to increased tissue catabolism. Frusemide is potentially nephrotoxic in large doses but does not cause hyperuraemia *per se*. However, hyperuricaemia and gout may occur. Captopril, like all ACE inhibitors, will result in renal impairment in renal artery stenosis. It will not, however, result in renal impairment in normal kidneys. ACE inhibitors are in fact beneficial in diabetic patients with early diabetic nephropathy (microalbuminuria). Spironolactone, a potassium-sparing diuretic (antagonising aldosterone) may result in hyperkalaemia but not increase plasma urea.

Ref: W McCaughey, R S J Clarke, J P H Fee, W F M Wallace. Anaesthetic Physiology and Pharmacology, 1st ed. Churchill Livingstone, 1997.

QUESTION 15

A. TRUE B. TRUE C. TRUE D. FALSE E. TRUE

Protamine is used to counteract the effect of heparin.

Antagonistic interactions may be classified into the following four categories:-

Competitive: The drugs bind reversibly and interaction is overcome by increasing the concentration of the agonist.
Irreversible (non-competitive): The drugs bind irreversibly (usually covalent bonding) and this cannot be overcome by increasing the concentration of the agonist.
Physiological: The interaction of two drugs whose opposing actions tend to cancel each other. e.g. noradrenaline increasing blood pressure and histamine decreasing blood pressure.
Chemical: Direct interaction of two drugs which either removes or prevents the drug from reaching the target. e.g. chelation of lead by penicillamine.

Ref: W McCaughey, R S J Clarke, J P H Fee, W F M Wallace. Anaesthetic Physiology and Pharmacology, 1st ed. Churchill Livingstone, 1997.

QUESTION 16

A. TRUE   B. FALSE   C. TRUE   D. FALSE   E. TRUE

All of the currently available non-depolarising muscle relaxants can be divided into two groups; aminosteroids and benzylisoquiniliniums.

Aminosteroids	Benzylisoquiniliniums
Pancuronium	Tubocurorarine
Pipercuronium	Atracurium
Vecuronium	Doxacurium
Rocuronium	Mivacurium

Ref: A R Aitkenhead, G Smith. Textbook of Anaesthesia, 3rd ed. Churchill Livingstone, 1996.

QUESTION 17

A. FALSE B. FALSE C. TRUE D. TRUE E. TRUE

The duration of action of oral frusemide is approximately 6 hours. The proprietary name for frusemide is Lasix and it is said to be so named because it last six hours.

In patients with renal impairment, larger doses may be needed. Frusemide may cause hyponatraemia, hypokalaemia, hypomagnesaemia, hyperuricaemia, hyperglycaemia, hypochloraemic alkalosis, increase in plasma cholesterol and triglyceride concentrations.

Ref: W McCaughey, R S J Clarke, J P H Fee, W F M Wallace. Anaesthetic Physiology and Pharmacology, 1st ed. Churchill Livingstone, 1997.

QUESTION 18

A. FALSE   B. TRUE   C. FALSE   D. TRUE   E. FALSE

Dantrolene is given by rapid intravenous injection, 1 mg/kg, repeated as required to a cumulative max of 10 mg/kg. Dantrium contains 3 g mannitol in each 20 mg vial. Hypotension, myocardial depression and hyperkalaemia have been reported with intravenous dantrolene and verapamil. Dantrolene *per se* will not cause hyperkalaemia, although hyperkalaemia is a common finding in malignant hyperthermia.

Ref: British National Formulary, 1997

QUESTION 19

A. FALSE   B. FALSE   C. TRUE   D. TRUE   E. TRUE

The action of non-depolarising muscle relaxant is prolonged by hypokalaemia, hypocalcaemia, hypermagnesaemia, and concurrent treatment with lithium and aminoglycosides.

Ref: W McCaughey, R S J Clarke, J P H Fee, W F M Wallace. Anaesthetic Physiology and Pharmacology, 1st ed. Churchill Livingstone, 1997.

QUESTION 20

A. FALSE B. FALSE C. TRUE D. TRUE E. TRUE

The apparent Vd is obtained by dividing the total dose by the blood concentration. A highly lipid-soluble drug will accumulate in the fatty tissues with very little of the original dose remaining in the blood, resulting in a large Vd. Digoxin distributes widely in muscles, heart, liver and fatty tissues. Warfarin which is highly bound to plasma proteins (99%), has a small apparent Vd because a higher proportion of the total dose remains in the plasma. Highly polar drugs, e.g. muscle relaxants and gentamicin will have a Vd very similar to the ECF volume (~15 litres).

Approximate volume of distribution in a 70 kg adult is:-

	Litres
Warfarin	7
Atracurium	12
Vecuronium	15
Gentamicin	18
Alfentanil	25
Thiopentone	160
Morphine	230
Fentanyl	250
Digoxin	600

Ref: W McCaughey, R S J Clarke, J P H Fee, W F M Wallace. Anaesthetic Physiology and Pharmacology, 1st ed. Churchill Livingstone, 1997.

QUESTION 21

A. TRUE B. TRUE C. TRUE D. TRUE E. TRUE

The rate of gastric emptying is proportional to the volume of the stomach contents, with approximately 1-3% of the total gastric content reaching the duodenum per minute at an exponential rate. The presence of fat, acid or hypertonic solutions in the duodenum initiates a neurally mediated inhibitory enterogastric reflex, delaying the rate of gastric emptying. Gastric emptying is also under the control of the autonomic nervous system. Increased vagal tone hastens gastric emptying. Anti-muscarinic agents therefore delay gastric emptying. Fear, anxiety and pain decrease gastric emptying.

Ref: W F Ganong. Review of Medical Physiology, 18th ed. Lange, 1997.

QUESTION 22

A. FALSE B. TRUE C. TRUE D. TRUE E. TRUE

Solution	pH
5% glucose in water	4.0
4% glucose in 0.18% saline	4.0
0.9% saline	6.0
Hartmanns	6.5
Haemaccel	7.3
Gelofusine	7.4
Sodium bicarbonate 8.4%	7.8

Ref: A R Aitkenhead, G Smith. Textbook of Anaesthesia, 3rd ed. Churchill Livingstone, 1996.

QUESTION 23

A. FALSE B. TRUE C. FALSE D. FALSE E. TRUE

The less elastic arteries in the elderly result in a rise in arterial pressure, especially systolic pressure. There is reduced body water, which affects the volume of distribution of some drugs. Reduction in plasma proteins is not uncommon in the elderly. There is an increase in sensitivity to some drugs and a reduction in anaesthetic requirements (MAC) with age. The functional residual capacity increases with age, but is less than the increase in closing volume. Therefore, the increase in closing volume may exceed the FRC. Vital capacity drops and residual volume increases. Glomerular filtration rate decreases 1% per year after the age of 40 years.

Ref: R S Atkinson, G B Rushman, N J H Davies. Lees Synopsis of Anaesthesia, 11th ed. Butterworth-Heinemann, 1993.

QUESTION 24

A. TRUE B. TRUE C. TRUE D. FALSE E. FALSE

Possible harmful effects of PEEP include:–

- Increased airway pressure and risk of barotrauma
- Reduction of cardiac output secondary to decreased venous return to the heart
- Rise in cerebral venous and intracranial pressures in parallel with increase in mean intrathoracic pressure
- There is decreased urine output as a consequence of increased ADH secretion

Ref: R S Atkinson, G B Rushman, N J H Davies. Lees Synopsis of Anaesthesia, 11th ed. Butterworth-Heinemann, 1993.

QUESTION 25

A. FALSE B. TRUE C. TRUE D. FALSE E. FALSE

Glutamate and aspartate are the major excitatory transmitters in the CNS. Glycine and GABA are inhibitory transmitters in the CNS.

QUESTION 26

A. FALSE B. TRUE C. FALSE D. FALSE E. FALSE

Changes in CPD blood with storage time

Test	Day			
	1	**7**	**14**	**21**
Blood pH	7.1	7.0	7.0	6.9
Blood pCO_2 (kPa)	6.4	10.7	14.7	18.7
Blood lactate (mmol/l)	41	101	145	179
Plasma HCO_3^- (mmol/l)	18	15	12	11
Plasma K^+ (mmol/l)	3.9	12	17	21
Plasma dextrose (mg/dl)	345	312	282	231
Plasma Hb (mg/dl)	1.7	7.8	13	19
2,3-DPG (μM/ml)	4.8	1.2	1.0	<1.0
Platelets (%)	10	0	0	0
Factors V and VIII (%)	70	50	40	20

QUESTION 27

A. FALSE B. FALSE C. FALSE D. FALSE E. FALSE

CSF is clear and colourless, has a pH of 7.33 and does not turn litmus paper pink.

The following may be used to identify CSF after a suspected dural tap:-

- CSF is warm when it falls on to the skin
- CSF forms a cloudy precipitate when it falls into 2.5% thiopentone
- The glucose contained in CSF will show up in a test strip

Ref: A R Aitkenhead, G Smith. Textbook of Anaesthesia, 3rd ed. Churchill Livingstone, 1996.

QUESTION 28

A. TRUE B. TRUE C. TRUE D. TRUE E. TRUE

Renin is released by the juxta-glomerular cells. Angiotensinogen, an α-2 globulin is produced in the liver. Renin splits angiotensinogen to angiotensin I which is converted by ACE in the lungs to Angiotensin II. Antagonism of Angiotensin II results in hypotension.

Losartan (Cozaar) is the first Angiotensin II antagonist used for hypertension. Aldosterone is produced from zona glomerulosa of the adrenal cortex.

Ref: W F Ganong. Review of Medical Physiology, 18th ed. Lange, 1997.

QUESTION 29

A. FALSE   B. TRUE   C. FALSE   D. TRUE   E. TRUE

Vasopressin (ADH) secretion is increased by hypovolaemia and in response to an increased in plasma osmolality. The secretion of ADH is higher during the night than the day. ADH acts by increasing the formation of cyclic-AMP in the collecting duct cells, increasing its permeability to water.

Ref: W F Ganong. Review of Medical Physiology, 18th ed. Lange, 1997.

QUESTION 30

A. TRUE   B. TRUE   C. TRUE   D. TRUE   E. FALSE

The 5 counter-regulatory hormones that antagonise the insulin-induced hypoglycaemia are adrenaline, noradrenaline, glucagon, growth hormone and cortisol. Insulin promotes protein anabolism, glycogen synthesis and deposition of fat. Insulin facilitates the passage of potassium ions into cells.

Ref: W F Ganong. Review of Medical Physiology, 18th ed. Lange, 1997.

QUESTION 31

A. TRUE   B. FALSE   C. FALSE   D. FALSE   E. FALSE

The adrenal medulla constitutes approximately 25% of the mass of the adrenal gland. The cell types can be distinguished morphologically - 90% of the cells are the adrenaline-secreting type which have large, less dense granules, and 10% are the noradrenaline-secreting type which have smaller, very dense granules.

Ref: W F Ganong. Review of Medical Physiology, 18th ed. Lange, 1997.

QUESTION 32

A. TRUE   B. TRUE   C. TRUE   D. FALSE   E. FALSE

Lung surfactant reduces surface tension at the air-liquid interface in the alveolus and small airways, thereby improving lung compliance, promoting alveolar stability, and reducing the tendency toward atelectasis at low lung volumes. Surfactants may also play a role in maintaining lung fluid balance.

Ref: J B West. Respiratory Physiology - the essentials, 5th ed. Williams and Wilkins, 1995.

QUESTION 33

A. FALSE B. TRUE C. FALSE D. FALSE E. FALSE

Methaemoglobinaemia is formed when the ferrous ion haem is converted to the ferric form. In sickle-cell trait, there is substitution of glutamine for valine in the sixth position on the ß-chain. In ß-thalasaemia, no ß-chains are produced or production is impaired.

Hereditary spherocytosis is inherited in an autosomal dominant manner. The red blood cell membrane has a defect in the structural protein, spectrin which results in the membrane becoming more permeable to Na^+ ions. This causes the cells to become spherical and more fragile.

Glucose-6-phophate dehydrogenase deficiency holds a vital position in the hexose monophosphate shunt. It is inherited in an X-linked manner. Haemolysis of red blood cell is triggered by infections, ingestion of fava beans and various drugs.

Ref: A R Aitkenhead, G Smith. Textbook of Anaesthesia, 3rd ed. Churchill Livingstone, 1996.

QUESTION 34

A. TRUE B. TRUE C. TRUE D. TRUE E. TRUE

Increased blood urea:-
High protein diet
Dehydration
Increased catabolism (surgery, trauma, infection)
Steroid therapy
Tetracycline therapy
Dehydration
Renal disease

Decreased blood urea:-
Old age
Low protein diet
Pregnancy (increased GFR)

QUESTION 35

A. TRUE B. TRUE C. FALSE D. TRUE E. TRUE

Raised serum alkaline phosphatase:-

Obstructive jaundice
Pagets disease
Osteomalacia
Adolescence
Pregnancy

QUESTION 36

A. FALSE B. FALSE C. TRUE D. FALSE E. FALSE

Blood glucose level is usually maintained in the first 24 hours. The body relies on the breakdown of hepatic glycogen to glucose for energy. Hepatic glycogen stores are small and therefore gluconeogenesis is soon necessary to maintain glucose levels. Gluconeogenesis takes place mainly from lactate, glycerol and amino acids (mainly alanine and glutamine). Lipolysis, the breakdown of the body's fat store, also occurs. Central nervous metabolism changes from glucose as a substrate to ketone bodies (derived from fatty acid oxidation in the liver), which now becomes the main source of energy.

Ref: W F Ganong. Review of Medical Physiology, 18th ed. Lange, 1997.

QUESTION 37

A. TRUE B. FALSE C. FALSE D. FALSE E. TRUE

Adipose tissue is an efficient way of storing energy and is the major source of fuel available, apart from muscle protein, in the long-term fasting state. Carbohydrate stores are small, consisting of glycogen in the liver and a small amount of circulatory glucose. The average daily energy intake of a 70 kg man is 2700 kcal (approx. 12000 kJ). These calories are normally provided as approximately:-

    320 kcal (1360 kJ) of protein (80g)
    200 kcal (4800 kJ) of carbohydrate (300g)
    1125 kcal (4625 kJ) of fat (125g)

Linoleic acid, from which arachidonic acid is derived, is an essential fatty acid.

Ref: W F Ganong. Review of Medical Physiology, 18th ed. Lange, 1997.

QUESTION 38

A. TRUE B. TRUE C. TRUE D. FALSE E. FALSE

The quite substantial decrease in FRC (up to 500 ml at term) together with the increase in tidal volume, results in relatively large volumes of inspired air mixing with smaller volumes of air in the lungs. Consequently, the composition of alveolar mixture can be altered rapidly. In addition, the pregnant woman has increased oxygen consumption and therefore hypoxia will develop more rapidly during apnoea, respiratory obstruction or breathing of hypoxic gas mixture. Airway resistance is decreased secondary to progesterone induced bronchial dilatation.

Ref: R D Miller. Anesthesia, 4th ed. Churchill Livingstone, 1994.

QUESTION 39

A. FALSE B. TRUE C. TRUE D. TRUE E. FALSE

The neonate has a compliant chest wall but a lower lung compliance than that of an adult. An increase in cardiac output is usually achieved by increasing heart rate and not stroke volume. Neonates have a higher metabolic rate than adults. The blood volume of a neonate is approximately 85 ml/kg.

Ref: A R Aitkenhead, G Smith. Textbook of Anaesthesia, 3rd ed. Churchill Livingstone, 1996.

QUESTION 40

A. TRUE B. TRUE C. TRUE D. TRUE E. TRUE

The earliest change of hyperkalaemia is the development of tall tented T waves. As plasma K^+ increases other changes include prolonged PR interval, shortened QT interval, widened QRS complexes and reduced P wave. The widened QRS complexes finally merge into the T waves resulting in a sine wave pattern. Further increases in K^+ (>10 mmol/l) results in ventricular fibrillation.

Ref: A R Aitkenhead, G Smith. Textbook of Anaesthesia, 3rd ed. Churchill Livingstone, 1996.

QUESTION 41

A. TRUE B. TRUE C. TRUE D. TRUE E. FALSE

Oxygen consumption = CI $\times$ (CaO_2 - CvO_2) $\times$ 10
Units: $ml/min/m^2$
Normal range: 100 - 180

CaO_2 = arterial oxygen content
($Hb \times SaO_2 \times 1.34$) + ($PaO_2 \times 0.003$)

CvO_2 = mixed venous oxygen content
($Hb \times SvO_2 \times 1.34$) + ($PvO_2 \times 0.003$)

QUESTION 42

A. FALSE B. TRUE C. TRUE D. TRUE E. TRUE

It is assumed that pulmonary capillary wedge pressure approximates to left atrial pressure, which in turn approximates to left ventricular end-diastolic volume. This is true in most circumstances. The position of the catheter tip must be in West's zone III portion of the lung (i.e. PAP > LAP > alveolar pressure; flow is independent of alveolar pressure). In the ventilated patient, alveolar pressure is raised and the boundary between zone III and zone II (i.e. PAP > alveolar pressure > LAP) will shift. This also occurs with lung disease.

QUESTION 43

A. TRUE B. TRUE C. TRUE D. TRUE E. TRUE

All of these conditions can cause inaccuracies in the thermodilution cardiac output measurements.

QUESTION 44

A. FALSE B. FALSE C. TRUE D. TRUE E. TRUE

A paramagnetic gas analyser is used to measure oxygen concentration. Halothane, and not isoflurane, can be measured using an ultraviolet gas analyser. In the Raman spectrometer, a beam of laser light is scattered by the gas molecules. The photon gives up a portion of its energy to the gas molecule and is re-emitted with a longer wavelength and shifted frequency, which is unique to the gas concerned. Thus the frequency components present in scattered light permit identification of the gas molecule present, whilst the amplitude of the peaks provides an indication of the concentrations of each gas. Photoacoustic spectroscopy is based on absorption by the gas of infrared radiation. It is used to measure nitrous oxide, carbon dioxide and anaesthetic agents. Mass spectrometers are capable of separating the components of complex gas mixtures according to their mass and charge by deflecting the charged ions in a magnetic field.

Ref: M K Sykes, M D Vickers, C J Hull. Principles of Measurement and Monitoring in Anaesthesia and Intensive Care, 3rd ed. Blackwell, 1991.

QUESTION 45

A. FALSE B. TRUE C. TRUE D. TRUE E. TRUE

The two glass spheres are filled with a weakly diamagnetic gas such as nitrogen. Paramagnetic analysers are affected by the presence of high concentrations of a diamagnetic background gas such as nitrous oxide and carbon dioxide. Another source of error is the presence of water vapour in the gas to be analysed.

Ref: M K Sykes, M D Vickers, C J Hull. Principles of Measurement and Monitoring in Anaesthesia and Intensive Care, 3rd ed. Blackwell, 1991.

QUESTION 46

A. FALSE B. TRUE C. FALSE D. FALSE E. FALSE

PCWP remains normal in ARDS, pulmonary hypertension, pulmonary embolus and tricuspid regurgitation.

QUESTION 47

A. FALSE B. FALSE C. TRUE D. TRUE E. TRUE

The non-return pressure relief valve is situated downstream of the vaporisers either on the back bar or near the common gas outlet. Its non-return design helps to prevent back pressure effects commonly encountered when using minute volume divider ventilators. The valve opens when the pressure in the back bar exceeds about 35 kPa. It's function is to protect the flowmeter and vaporiser components, and not the patient.

The emergency oxygen flush allows an oxygen flow of about 45 l/min at a pressure of about 400 kPa. It should not be activated while ventilating a patient using a minute volume divider ventilator. Inappropriate use of the emergency oxygen flush leads to dilution of the anaesthetic gases and possible awareness.

In the UK, the oxygen control knob for the flowmeter is traditionally situated to the left. A crack in a flowmeter may result in a hypoxic mixture. To avoid this, oxygen is the last gas to be added to the mixture delivered to the back bar.

Ref: B Al-Shaikh, S Stacey. Essentials of Anaesthetic Equipment, Churchill Livingstone, 1995.

QUESTION 48

A. FALSE B. FALSE C. TRUE D. FALSE E. FALSE

Cylinders are made of lightweight molybdenum steel (an alloy of steel and chromium) to withstand high pressure, e.g. 13,700 kPa for oxygen. The year when the cylinder was last examined can be identified from the shape and colour of the disc. The body and shoulder of the cylinder are colour-coded to identify the gas it contains. The cylinders attached to the anaesthetic machine are usually size E. The filling ratio is the weight of the fluid in the cylinder divided by the weight of water required to fill the cylinder. In the UK, the filling ratio for nitrous oxide is 0.75. Tare weight is the weight of the cylinder when empty.

Ref: B Al-Shaikh, S Stacey. Essentials of Anaesthetic Equipment, Churchill Livingstone, 1995.

QUESTION 49

A. FALSE B. FALSE C. TRUE D. FALSE E. TRUE

The Tec 6 design is completely different from the previous Tec series but can be mounted on the Selectatec system without the use of a special adaptor.

Desflurane has a saturated vapour pressure of 664 mmHg at 20°C and a boiling point of 23.5°C at atmospheric pressure. In order to overcome these physical properties, the vaporisation chamber is heated to a temperature of 39°C with a pressure of 1,550 mmHg (approximately 2 bar).

The dial calibration is from 0–18% with 1% graduations from 0–10% and 2% graduations from 10–18%.

A fixed restriction is positioned in the fresh gas flow path. The fresh gas flow does not enter the vaporisation chamber.

Ref: B Al-Shaikh, S Stacey. Essentials of Anaesthetic Equipment, Churchill Livingstone, 1995.

QUESTION 50

A. FALSE B. FALSE C. FALSE D. TRUE E. TRUE

The Cardiff Aldasorber contains charcoal granules used to absorb halogenated inhalational agents, but not nitrous oxide or carbon dioxide. The increase in weight of the canister is the only indication that it is exhausted. Heating the canister causes the release of the inhalational agents.

Ref: B Al-Shaikh, S Stacey. Essentials of Anaesthetic Equipment, Churchill Livingstone, 1995.

QUESTION 51

A. TRUE B. FALSE C. TRUE D. TRUE E. TRUE

In order to measure arterial blood gases, a sample of heparinised, anaerobic and fresh blood is needed. Heparin is added to the sample to prevent clotting during analysis. The heparin should only fill the dead space of the syringe and form a thin film on its interior. Excess heparin, which is acidic, lowers the pH of the sample. The presence of air bubbles increases the PaO_2 and decreases the $PaCO_2$.

An old blood sample has a lower pH and PaO_2, and a higher $PaCO_2$. If there is a need to delay analysis, the sample should be kept on ice.

The measured parameters are: pH, PaO_2 and $PaCO_2$.
The derived parameters are: actual bicarbonate, standard bicarbonate, base excess and SaO_2.

Ref: B Al-Shaikh, S Stacey. Essentials of Anaesthetic Equipment, Churchill Livingstone, 1995.

QUESTION 52

A. FALSE B. TRUE C. FALSE D. FALSE E. FALSE

The saturated vapour pressure of a volatile agent is dependent on the ambient temperature. It is not dependent on the atmospheric pressure. The volume and surface area of the liquid will affect the rate of vaporisation but once equilibrium is reached, the SVP remains the same at the same ambient temperature. The composition of the different gases will not alter the partial pressure of the volatile liquid at the ambient temperature and pressure because the SVP will remain the same. However, according to Dalton's law, the partial pressure of the other gases will change accordingly when the composition of the gases is altered.

Ref: P D Davis, G D Parbrook, G N C Kenny. Basic Physics and Measurement in Anaesthesia, 4th ed. Butterworth-Heinemann, 1995.

QUESTION 53

A. TRUE   B. TRUE   C. FALSE   D. TRUE   E. TRUE

Although mass spectrometers and gas analysers based on Raman scattering can measure the concentration of expired CO_2, the infrared absorption technique is most popular. This method involves passing infrared light of a particular wavelength (4,300 nm or 4.3 micrometre) through a very small amount of expired gas. CO_2 then absorbs the infrared light in proportion to the concentration of CO_2. As with other absorption spectrophotometers, the function of the infrared CO_2 analyser is based on the Beer-Lambert law. The windows on the chambers are made of sapphire, because glass would absorb infrared light. Infrared light may be absorbed by any molecule that is both asymmetric and polyatomic. Therefore single atoms such as helium, argon and hydrogen and symmetric molecules, such as O_2 and N_2, will not absorb infrared light. Asymmetric molecules such as CO_2, water vapour, nitrous oxide and anaesthetic agents will absorb infrared light. The infrared absorption peaks for some of these molecules, especially nitrous oxide, overlap with the absorption peaks of CO_2. To correct for this interference by nitrous oxide, it is necessary to use an additional wavelength of light to measure the concentration of nitrous oxide independently (i.e. 3,900 nm). A second process known as collision broadening can also interfere with the infrared absorption by CO_2. Collision broadening interference is most significant for nitrous oxide, O_2 and N_2. Capnometers incorporate corrections for nitrous oxide and O_2 in the gas mixture.

Ref: R D Miller. Anesthesia, 4th ed. Churchill Livingstone, 1994.

QUESTION 54

A. FALSE   B. FALSE   C. TRUE   D. TRUE   E. TRUE

Capnography, the measurement of CO_2 in expired gases, is undertaken using infrared absorption, mass spectrometry and Raman analysis. The majority of capnographs rely on infrared absorption.

Clark electrode and paramagnetic analyser are used for measuring oxygen tension.

Ref: R D Miller. Anesthesia, 4th ed. Churchill Livingstone, 1994.

QUESTION 55

A. TRUE   B. FALSE   C. TRUE   D. FALSE   E. TRUE

The P wave is produced by atrial depolarisation, the QRS complex by ventricular depolarisation. The PR interval starts from the beginning of the P wave and ends at the begining of the QRS complex. Repolarisation of the ventricles begins at the end of the QRS complex and consists of the ST segment and T wave. The T wave represents the uncancelled potential differences of ventricular repolarisation.

Ref: R D Miller. Anesthesia, 4th ed. Churchill Livingstone, 1994.

QUESTION 56

A. FALSE B. FALSE C. TRUE D. TRUE E. TRUE

In 1956, Clark developed the polarographic oxygen electrode for measuring oxygen partial pressure. With the development of the Severinghaus CO_2 electrode in 1958, the blood gas machine was developed. The Clark electrode is an electrical cell composed of a platinum cathode and a silver anode. As in any resistive circuit, as the voltage is increased the current will also increase. In this electrochemical cell there is a plateau voltage range over which the current does not increase with voltage but does increase with oxygen tension in the cell. A voltage of 0.6 V is applied between its electrodes. This is in contrast to a fuel cell which does not require a voltage.

An oxygen consuming electrochemical reaction takes place at the cathode, and the electric current in the circuit is directly proportional to the oxygen consumed at the cathode. The reaction is temperature sensitive. The cell is covered with a membrane which is freely permeable to oxygen. Clark's polarographic oxygen electrode has been used for over 30 years to measure oxygen partial pressure in gases and liquids.

Ref: K K Tremper, T W Rutter, J A Wahr. Monitoring Oxygenation. Current Anaesthesia and Critical Care 1993; 4: 213-222.

QUESTION 57

A. FALSE B. TRUE C. FALSE D. TRUE E. TRUE

The risk of ventricular fibrillation is greatest if the AC current has a frequency of 50 Hz. High frequency currents (0.3-3 MHz) are used to minimise the danger of excitation of cardiac muscle. High frequency continuous oscillation is used for cutting, while bursts of lower frequency are preferred for coagulation.

In a monopolar diathermy, current flows between the active electrode and the plate (indifferent) electrode. The active electrode should make only a small area of contact with the tissue so the current density is high and direct heating of the tissue occurs. The plate (indifferent) electrode makes a large area of contact with the patient and the current density is low, so that no tissue damage occurs. Diathermy burns may occur under the plate electrode if the plate makes poor contact with the patient (the small area of contact results in a high current density and a burn may result at this point). Poor plate contact is likely to raise the impedance of the circuit. Thus the machine will not perform satisfactorily at its usual setting and the output of the generator will have to be increased. This should alert theatre staff to the possibility of a badly connected plate. Another danger of the high impedance of the plate electrode is that the current may then be able to pass to earth via an alternative route, such as ECG electrodes or tracheal tubes. Since these have small areas of contact and therefore a high current density, there is consequently a risk of burning.

Bipolar diathermy relies on the passage of current between two electrodes close together thus minimising the passage of current through the body, so avoiding risks associated with pacemakers.

Ref: C Scurr, S Feldman, N Soni. Scientific Foundations of Anaesthesia, 4th ed. Heinemann, 1990.

QUESTION 58

A. TRUE B. TRUE   C. TRUE   D. TRUE   E. FALSE

External defibrillation of the heart involves the delivery of an adequate electrical current flow through the heart, via electrodes applied to the chest wall, causing simultaneous depolarisation of all myocardial cells that are at that moment fully refractory. Defibrillators consist of a power source (battery, AC source), voltage selector, AC-DC converter, capacitor and electrodes. The output energy of the defibrillation pulse is usually expressed in joules, where:

Energy (Joules) = Power (W) × duration (s)

and

Power = Potential × Current *and* Current = Potential ÷ Impedance.

The amount of current flowing through the heart depends on the energy of the shock and, transthoracic impedance.

Transthoracic impedance depends on many factors:-
 - time to defibrillation
 - previous shocks
 - ventilatory phase
 - electrode size, contact, pressure and distance from the heart

Larger electrode pads are associated with a lower transthoracic impedance and improved defibrillation success rates with low energy shocks. The optimum size is approximately 13 cm in diameter in adults.

The output waveform of most conventional external defibrillators is half sinusoidal (damped Edmark waveform). The optimum duration of the waveform is 4-12 ms.

Inspired by the experience of implanted automatic defibrillators, the use of biphasic or triphasic waveforms is being investigated. Using these waveforms, the defibrillation threshold seems to be lower and there may be less functional and morphological damage to the myocardium.

Ref: L L Bossaert. Fibrillation and defibrillation of the heart. British Journal of Anaesthesia 1997; 79: 203-213.

QUESTION 59

A. TRUE   B. TRUE   C. TRUE   D. TRUE   E. FALSE

As the critical temperature of nitrous oxide is well above room temperature (36.5° C), this gas may be stored in cylinders as a liquid. Nitrous oxide is stored in compressed form as a liquid in cylinders at a pressure of 50 bar (5,000 kPa). Because the cylinder contains liquid and vapour, the total quantity of nitrous oxide contained in a cylinder can be ascertained only by weighing.

If a full cylinder is allowed to empty slowly (say at a flow rate of 100 ml/min), the liquid draws heat from the surroundings rapidly enough to remain at room temperature, and the indicated pressure remains unchanged until the last drop of liquid is evaporated. The pressure then falls in accordance with Boyle's law until it is equal to the ambient pressure.

At a higher flow rate (e.g. 6 l/min) the liquid cannot gain heat from the surroundings rapidly enough to remain at room temperature. Ice may be seen to form at the foot of the cylinder. As the liquid cools there is a corresponding reduction in SVP and, therefore, the indicated pressure.

Ref: W S Nimmo, G Smith. Anaesthesia, 2nd ed. Blackwell, 1994.

QUESTION 60

A. FALSE   B. TRUE   C. TRUE   D. TRUE   E. FALSE

Compliance is a measure of the change in lung volume per unit change in airway pressure. Compliance is a static measure of lung and chest recoil. Compliance depends on lung volume and a patient with only one lung has approximately half the change in volume for a given change in airway pressure. Compliance is slightly greater when measured during deflation than when measured during inflation. Compliance is increased in emphysema and decreased in pulmonary oedema and interstitial pulmonary fibrosis

Ref: W F Ganong. Review of Medical Physiology, 18th ed. Lange, 1997.

Exam 5

QUESTION 1

The following drugs have an elimination half-life of greater than 3 hours

A. Amiodarone
B. Thiopentone
C. Propofol
D. Fentanyl
E. Alfentanil

QUESTION 2

The following drugs readily cross the normal blood–brain barrier

A. Benzylpenicillin
B. Physostigmine
C. Neostigmine
D. Glycopyrollate
E. Vecuronium

QUESTION 3

Drugs which may cause a decrease in serum potassium concentration include

A. Insulin
B. Frusemide
C. Digoxin
D. Theophylline
E. Calcium antagonist

QUESTION 4

The following antibiotics are bacteriostatic

A. Gentamicin
B. Cefuroxime
C. Erythromycin
D. Tetracycline
E. Vancomycin

QUESTION 5

The following antifungal agents are suitable for candida infection

A. Nystatin
B. Griseofulvin
C. Ketoconazole
D. Fluconazole
E. Amphotericin

QUESTION 6

The following are negative inotropes

A. Nifedipine
B. Lisinopril
C. Amiodarone
D. Glucagon
E. Atenolol

QUESTION 7

The following drugs are antagonised by naloxone

A. Dextropropoxyphene
B. Midazolam
C. Buprenorphine
D. Remifentanil
E. Thiopentone

QUESTION 8

Drugs promoting gastric emptying include

A. Metoclopramide
B. Domperidone
C. Cisapride
D. Sucralfate
E. Nizatidine

QUESTION 9

Drugs to be avoided in heart failure include

A. Verapamil
B. Atenolol
C. Lisinopril
D. Enalapril
E. Glyceryl trinitrate

QUESTION 10

Drugs suitable for supraventricular arrhythmias include

A. Adenosine
B. Verapamil
C. Bretylium
D. Lignocaine
E. Amiodarone

QUESTION 11

Drugs suitable for ventricular arrhythmias include

A. Flecainide
B. Phenytoin
C. Mexiletine
D. Disopyramide
E. Digoxin

QUESTION 12

Drugs suitable for both supraventricular and ventricular arrhythmias include

A. Amiodarone
B. Procainamide
C. Propafenone
D. Flecainide
E. Digoxin

QUESTION 13

The following drugs are 5-HT agonists

A. Ondansetron
B. Granisetron
C. Selegiline
D. Sumatriptan
E. Lamotrigine

QUESTION 14

Antibiotics which are bactericidal

A. Penicillins
B. Aminoglycosides
C. Vancomycin
D. Erythromycin
E. Metronidazole

QUESTION 15

Advantages of ACTH over prednisolone include a lower incidence of

A. Acne
B. Fluid retention
C. Osteoporosis
D. Growth retardation in children
E. Adrenal insufficiency with intercurrent stress

QUESTION 16

Metronidazole is active against

A. Giardia lamblia
B. Bacteroides fragilis
C. Entamoeba histolytica
D. Clostridium welchii
E. Actinomyces

QUESTION 17

Pulmonary fibrosis is an unwanted side-effect of

A. Amiodarone
B. Bleomycin
C. Digoxin
D. Nitrofurantoin
E. Busulphan

QUESTION 18

Uterine tone is reduced by

A. Ritodrine
B. Vecuronium
C. Ketamine
D. Isoflurane
E. Salbutamol

QUESTION 19

The following are recognised side-effects of the drugs listed in brackets

A. Pancreatitis (Frusemide)
B. Nasal congestion (Phenoxybenzamine)
C. Cough (Enalapril)
D. Dry mouth (Cyclizine)
E. Increased bronchial secretion (Chlormethiazole)

QUESTION 20

Helium, when compared with nitrogen

A. Is less dense
B. Has a lower viscosity
C. Has a higher thermal conductivity
D. Has less narcotic effect
E. Diffuses more rapidly into the body tissues

QUESTION 21

Cyanosis

A. Occurs when blood contains over 5 g/dl of carbaminohaemoglobin
B. Can be produced by 1.5 g/dl of methaemoglobin
C. Is more readily detected in anaemia
D. Is common in carbon monoxide poisoning
E. Does not occur in histotoxic hypoxia

QUESTION 22

The Valsalva Manoeuvre

A. Is associated with an initial fall in arterial pressure at the onset of straining
B. Is associated with bradycardia during the manoeuvre
C. Causes stimulation of the baroreceptors during the manoeuvre
D. Results in increased intracranial pressure
E. Heart rate changes may be absent in diabetes mellitus

QUESTION 23

The carotid body

A. Consists of stretch receptors
B. Has a blood flow approximately four times that of the brain
C. Is stimulated by a decrease in pH
D. Is stimulated by carbon monoxide poisoning
E. Is stimulated by cyanide poisoning

QUESTION 24

Regarding body temperature control

A. The autonomic nervous system has an important role in thermoregulation
B. The pineal gland is the principal structure within the CNS co-ordinating thermoregulation
C. Cold and warm thermosensors exist in the skin
D. In neonates, brown fat is found predominantly around the thigh and buttocks
E. Brown fat metabolism is activated by the autonomic nervous system

QUESTION 25

The following sites have a good correlation with core temperature

A. Tympanic membrane
B. Lower oesophagus
C. Bladder
D. Rectum
E. Axilla

QUESTION 26

Cardiac muscle

A. Behaves as a syncytium
B. Does not contain troponin
C. Fibre consists of multiple nuclei
D. Fibres have a resting membrane potential of approximately - 60 mV
E. Action potentials last approximately 15 ms

QUESTION 27

The following are parasympathetic ganglia

A. Stellate ganglion
B. Coeliac ganglion
C. Ciliary ganglion
D. Otic ganglion
E. Gasserian ganglion

QUESTION 28

Stellate ganglion block causes

A. Ptosis
B. Miosis
C. Anhydrosis
D. Dilated conjunctival vessels
E. Nasal congestion

QUESTION 29

The following results points to hypovolaemia rather than acute tubular necrosis as the cause of the reduced urine output

A. Urine osmolality 600 mosmol/kg
B. Urine sodium 40 mmol/l
C. Urine : plasma creatinine ratio 10
D. Urine : plasma urea ratio 5
E. Urine : plasma osmolality ratio 1

QUESTION 30

Ventilation/perfusion ratio of less than 1.0 is associated with

A. Pneumonia
B. Hypovolaemic shock
C. Pulmonary oedema
D. Pulmonary embolus
E. Pulmonary contusion

QUESTION 31

At birth, the following are true

A. There is a marked decrease in pulmonary vascular resistance
B. The right ventricular wall is thicker than the left
C. The increased flow of blood to the left atrium causes the ductus arteriosus to close
D. The haemoglobin concentration is approximately 10 g/dl
E. Myelination of the nervous system is complete

QUESTION 32

The following factors predispose to pulmonary oedema

A. Low pulmonary capillary pressure
B. Decreased oncotic pressure
C. Increased capillary permeability
D. Impairment of lymphatic drainage
E. Rapid lung expansion

QUESTION 33

In vigorous exercise

A. Pulse pressure increases
B. Total peripheral resistance decreases
C. Respiratory quotient decreases
D. Skin blood flow decreases
E. Renal blood flow decreases

QUESTION 34

A child whose mother has blood group B and father has blood group A may have the following blood group genotype

A. OO
B. AA
C. BB
D. AB
E. OA

QUESTION 35

Parathyroid hormone

A. Is a polypeptide
B. Increases calcium absorption from the intestine
C. Increases synthesis of 24, 25-dihydroxycholecalciferol
D. Decreases plasma phosphate
E. Is increased in osteoporosis

QUESTION 36

Concerning the knee jerk

A. It is a monosynaptic reflex
B. The stimulus arises from the tendon
C. Impulses travel via Ia afferent fibres
D. The response is contraction of the quadriceps femoris muscle
E. The Golgi tendon organ is an important component

QUESTION 37

Smooth muscle cells

A. Have no cross-striations
B. Do not contain actin
C. Comprise multinucleated cells
D. Act as a syncytium
E. Are under somatic nervous control

QUESTION 38

Concerning skeletal muscle

A. It comprises multinucleated cells
B. The resting membrane potential is approximately - 60 mV
C. During contraction, the width of the A bands is reduced
D. During a complete tetanus, the tension developed is greater than that developed by an individual twitch contraction
E. It is innervated by the autonomic nervous system

QUESTION 39

The ideal substance for determining glomerular filtration rate

A. Has a molecular weight greater than 69,000
B. Is 100% bound to plasma proteins
C. Is freely filtered from the plasma
D. Is entirely reabsorbed in the tubules
E. Is actively secreted by tubules

QUESTION 40

Following total gastrectomy

A. Hypoglycaemia may occur
B. Hyperglycaemia may occur
C. Protein digestion is deficient
D. Iron deficiency may occur
E. Megaloblastic anaemia may occur

QUESTION 41

In an exponentially changing process

A. The rate of change of X is directly proportional to X
B. The relationship can be made linear by logarithmic transformation
C. One half-life is equal to approximately 70% of the time constant
D. The time constant is the time taken for the process to reach 36.8% of the starting value
E. After 2 time constants 86.5% of a process would have been completed if the initial rate of change had continued

QUESTION 42

The following are true regarding breathing systems

A. The Bain circuit is an example of a Mapleson A system
B. The Bain circuit is more efficient than the Lack circuit during spontaneous breathing
C. In the Bain circuit, fresh gas flow occurs through the outer tube
D. During spontaneous breathing, the Lack circuit requires a fresh gas flow rate of twice the alveolar minute ventilation to prevent rebreathing
E. The Lack circuit may be used to ventilate the patient's lungs with the Penlon Nuffield 200 ventilator

QUESTION 43

A standard 12 lead ECG in an asymptomatic patient

A. Showing right bundle branch block does not indicate heart disease
B. Showing left bundle branch block is an indication of heart disease
C. Showing the Mobitz type I heart block (Wenckebach) is an indicator for pacing
D. Showing an inverted T wave in VR may be due to lateral ischaemia
E. Showing sinus arrhythmia may indicate the presence of autonomic neuropathy

QUESTION 44

The following measurements are reliable and provide an early detection of air embolism

A. ECG
B. Pulse oximetry
C. Capnography
D. Precordial auscultation with stethoscope
E. Doppler ultrasound

QUESTION 45

Pressure-volume loops can be used to measure

A. Compliance
B. Functional residual capacity (FRC)
C. Work of breathing
D. Airway resistance
E. Closing volume

QUESTION 46

The following gases support combustion

A. Helium
B. Argon
C. Nitrous oxide
D. Carbon dioxide
E. Isoflurane

QUESTION 47

Concerning gas flow through a tube

A. For laminar flow, halving the radius decreases the flow 8-fold
B. Viscosity of the gas is a major determinant in turbulent flow
C. Reynold's number greater than 2,000 is more likely to result in turbulent flow
D. A gas with high density is likely to increase Reynold's number
E. A gas with high viscosity is likely to increase Reynold's number

QUESTION 48

The following statements are true

A. Turbulent flow is less likely with 70% nitrous oxide in oxygen than air
B. Helium has a lower density than nitrogen
C. Carbon dioxide when passed through a flowmeter calibrated for nitrous oxide will give accurate flow rates
D. The viscosity of a liquid increases with increase in temperature
E. The viscosity of a gas increases with increase in temperature

QUESTION 49

A passive scavenging system

A. Employs a device to generate a negative pressure within the system in order to expel waste gases
B. Should produce resistance to expiration of no greater than 0.5 cmH_2O (50 Pa) at a flow rate of 30 l/min
C. Has a positive pressure relief valve set to 10 cmH_2O (1,000 Pa)
D. Has a negative pressure relief valve set at -5 cmH_2O (-50 Pa)
E. May generate negative pressures under certain conditions

QUESTION 50

The following statements are true regarding monitoring of non–depolarising neuromuscular blockade

A. A post-tetanic count of 5 correlates with a train-of-four ratio of approximately 0.7
B. A post tetanic count of greater than 4 is generally considered suitable for extubation
C. When a patient is able to sustain head lift for 5 seconds, less than 70% of receptors will still be occupied by the neuromuscular blocker
D. ToF–Watch is a device for monitoring neuromuscular block by means of acceleromyogrophy
E. ToF–Guard is a device for monitoring neuromuscular block by means of a force transducer

QUESTION 51

Regarding the vaporisation of a liquid

A. The saturated vapour pressure (SVP) increases with temperature
B. The boiling point is the temperature at which its SVP becomes equal to the ambient pressure
C. At high altitude, the concentration of a saturated vapour is increased
D. At high altitude, the SVP is reduced
E. At the critical temperature, the energy required to vaporise the liquid is zero

QUESTION 52

The following exist as liquids at room temperature when stored in pressurised cylinders

A. Oxygen
B. Nitrous oxide
C. Entonox
D. Carbon dioxide
E. Air

QUESTION 53

In the constant pressure bobbin flowmeter (Rotameter)

A. Carbon dioxide will produce accurate readings if passed through a nitrous oxide flowmeter at low flow rates
B. Carbon dioxide will produce accurate readings if passed through a nitrous oxide flowmeter at high flow rates
C. Air will produce accurate readings if passed through a nitrous oxide flowmeter at low flow rates
D. Oxygen will produce accurate readings if passed through a carbon dioxide flowmeter at low flow rates
E. Oxygen will produce accurate readings if passed through a carbon dioxide flowmeter at high flow rates

QUESTION 54

The following describes an optimal arrangement for efficiency and economy in a circle absorber system

A. The fresh gas inlet is positioned in the inspired gas stream proximal to the inspiratory valve
B. Expired gas is vented via the overflow valve from the circuit upstream of the soda lime canister
C. The soda lime is positioned before the fresh gas inlet
D. The reservoir bag is positioned upstream of the soda lime
E. The overflow valve is positioned between the soda lime canister and fresh gas inlet

QUESTION 55

The following statements are true regarding monitoring of non-depolarising neuromuscular blockade

A. The duration of electrical stimulus in a single twitch is 2 ms
B. The intensity of a supramaximal stimulation is 100 mA for a surface electrode
C. The intensity of a supramaximal stimulation is 50 mA for a needle electrode
D. For a 50 Hz, 5 second tetanus, post-tetanic potentiation persists for at least 1 minute
E. Train-of-four stimulation can be repeated after 15 seconds

QUESTION 56

The following nerve/muscle combination may be used in the monitoring of neuromuscular blockade

A. Ulnar nerve/Abductor pollicis brevis
B. Ulnar nerve/Adductor pollicis
C. Ulnar nerve/Opponens pollicis
D. Facial nerve/Orbicularis oculi
E. Common peroneal nerve/Tibialis anterior

QUESTION 57

The following statements are true regarding the monitoring of non-depolarising neuromuscular blockade

A. The diaphragm is more sensitive than the tibialis anterior muscle
B. The orbicularis oculi is more sensitive than adductor pollicis
C. Adductor pollicis may still be paralysed, even after the patient has resumed normal respiration
D. Stimulation of the median nerve results in adduction of the thumb
E. Stimulation of the common peroneal nerve results in plantar flexion of the foot

QUESTION 58

The following statements are true regarding the monitoring of non-depolarising neuromuscular blockade

A. Onset of neuromuscular block is more rapid at the diaphragm than at the adductor pollicis
B. Intensity of block is less at the orbicularis oculi than at the adductor pollicis
C. In the train-of-four stimulation, the fourth evoked response is eliminated at about 75% depression of the control
D. T4/T1 ratio >75% is equivalent to being able to raise the head from the pillow and protrude the tongue on command
E. When the double-burst stimulation is used, determination of fade is possible when the train-of-four ratio is 0.5 or less

QUESTION 59

End-tidal CO_2

A. Can be measured using an infrared analyser
B. Is usually slightly greater than the $PaCO_2$
C. Reading decreases with air emboli
D. Reading decreases with pulmonary emboli
E. Reading increases with decreased cardiac output

QUESTION 60

The following conditions cause inaccuracies in pulse oximetry reading

A. Carbon monoxide poisoning
B. Haemoglobin S disease
C. Jaundice
D. Anaemia
E. Polycythaemia

Exam 5: Answers

QUESTION 1

A. TRUE B. TRUE C. TRUE D. TRUE E. FALSE

Amiodarone has an elimination half-life of days.
Thiopentone has an elimination half-life of 10 hrs.
Propofol has an elimination half-life of 4 hrs.
Fentanyl has an elimination half-life of 4 hrs.
Alfentanil has an elimination half-life of 1.5 hrs.

Ref: W McCaughey, R S J Clarke, J P H Fee, W F M Wallace. Anaesthetic Physiology and Pharmacology, 1st ed. Churchill Livingstone, 1997.

QUESTION 2

A. FALSE B. TRUE C. FALSE D. FALSE E. FALSE

The major feature of the blood-brain barrier is that it behaves mainly like a continuous lipid membrane. Drugs which are highly ionised, such as quaternary ammonium compounds, will not cross the blood-brain barrier readily. The permeability of the blood-brain barrier may be increased if the tight junctions between cells are opened up. This may occur in inflammation of the meninges (hence benzylpenicillin, although not able to cross the normal blood-brain barrier, can be used to treat meningitis). Other conditions where this blood-brain barrier may be more permeable include hypertensive encephalopathy, cerebral ischaemia or head injury.

Ref: W McCaughey, R S J Clarke, J P H Fee, W F M Wallace. Anaesthetic Physiology and Pharmacology, 1st ed. Churchill Livingstone, 1997.

QUESTION 3

A. TRUE B. TRUE C. FALSE D. TRUE E. FALSE

Insulin causes hypokalaemia by shifting serum potassium into the cells. Frusemide and bumetanide are loop diuretics, which may cause hypokalaemia, hyponatraemia, hypomagnesaemia, hypochloraemic alkalosis and increased calcium excretion. Digoxin does not have any effect on serum potassium but hypokalaemia increases the risk of digoxin toxicity. Potassium-sparing diuretics include amiloride, triamterene, spironolactone, and potassium canrenoate. Theophylline is capable of producing hypokalaemia, particularly in overdose. Calcium antagonist has no effect on serum potassium.

Ref: British National Formulary, 1997.

QUESTION 4

A. FALSE   B. FALSE   C. TRUE   D. TRUE   E. FALSE

Bactericidal:
    Aminoglycosides, Penicillins, Cephalosporins,
    Co-trimoxazole, Isoniazid, Metronidazole, Vancomycin

Bacteriostatic:
    Erythromycin, Sulphonamides, Tetracyclines

Ref: W McCaughey, R S J Clarke, J P H Fee, W F M Wallace. Anaesthetic Physiology and Pharmacology, 1st ed. Churchill Livingstone, 1997.

QUESTION 5

A. TRUE   B. FALSE   C. TRUE   D. TRUE   E. TRUE

Griseofulvin is selectively concentrated in keratin and is the drug of choice for dermatophyte infections. It is not active against yeasts and therefore not suitable for candida infections.

Ref: British National Formulary, 1997.

QUESTION 6

A. TRUE   B. FALSE   C. TRUE   D. FALSE   E. TRUE

Nifedipine should be avoided in heart failure as it depresses myocardial contractility. ACE inhibitors have a valuable role in all grades of heart failure and have been shown to improve prognosis. Amiodarone, particularly when given intravenously, can cause myocardial depression. Glucagon is a positive inotrope. All β-blockers slow the heart and may cause myocardial depression and precipitate heart failure.

Ref: W McCaughey, R S J Clarke, J P H Fee, W F M Wallace. Anaesthetic Physiology and Pharmacology, 1st ed. Churchill Livingstone, 1997.

QUESTION 7

A. TRUE   B. FALSE   C. TRUE   D. TRUE   E. FALSE

All opioids are antagonised by naloxone. Midazolam is a benzodiazepine and is antagonised by flumazenil. Thiopentone is a barbiturate and not antagonised by naloxone.

Ref: British National Formulary, 1997.

QUESTION   8

A. TRUE   B. TRUE   C. TRUE   D. FALSE   E. FALSE

Metoclopramide and domperidone are dopamine antagonists which stimulate gastric empty-ing and increase the lower oesophageal tone. Cisapride is a motility stimulant, promoting gastric emptying by releasing ACh in the gut wall. Sucralfate is a complex of aluminium hydroxide and sulphated sucrose, used for the prophylaxis and treatment of peptic ulcers. It acts by protecting the gastric mucosa from acid–pepsin attack.

Nizatidine is one of the newer H2 receptor antagonists.

Ref: W McCaughey, R S J Clarke, J P H Fee, W F M Wallace. Anaesthetic Physiology and Pharmacology, 1st ed. Churchill Livingstone, 1997.

QUESTION   9

A. TRUE   B. TRUE   C. FALSE   D. FALSE   E. FALSE

Verapamil depresses myocardial function and may precipitate heart failure. Other calcium-channel blockers e.g. diltiazem, amlodipine and felodipine do not impair myocardial contrac-tility. All β-blockers may induce myocardial depression and precipitate heart failure.

Lisinopril and enalapril (ACE inhibitors) improve the prognosis of patients with heart failure. Nitrates cause a reduction in venous return, which reduces left ventricular work and are there-fore useful in the treatment of left ventricular failure.

Ref: British National Formulary, 1997.

QUESTION   10

A. TRUE   B. TRUE   C. FALSE   D. FALSE   E. TRUE

Drugs suitable for supraventricular arrhythmias:
   Adenosine
   Amiodarone
   Digoxin
   Disopyramide
   Flecainide
   Procainamide
   Propafenone
   Quinidine
   Verapamil

Ref: British National Formulary, 1997.

QUESTION 11

A. TRUE   B. TRUE   C. TRUE   D. TRUE   E. FALSE

Drugs suitable for ventricular arrhythmias:
Amiodarone
Bretylium
Disopyramide
Flecainide
Lignocaine
Mexiletine
Moracizine
Phenytoin
Procainamide
Propafenone
Quinidine
Tocainide

Ref: British National Formulary, 1997.

QUESTION 12

A. TRUE B. TRUE   C. TRUE   D. TRUE   E. FALSE

Drugs suitable for both supraventricular and ventricular arrhythmias:
Amiodarone
Disopyramide
Flecainide
Procainamide
Propafenone
Quinidine

Ref: British National Formulary, 1997.

QUESTION 13

A. FALSE   B. FALSE   C. FALSE   D. TRUE   E. FALSE

$5-HT_1$ agonists such as sumatriptan, zolmitriptan and naratriptan are used for migraine attacks. Ondansetron, granisetron and tropisetron are specific $5-HT_3$ antagonists. Selegiline is a monoamine–oxidase–B inhibitor used in severe parkinsonism in conjunction with levodopa to reduce end-of-dose deterioration. Lamotrigine is one of the newer antiepileptic agents.

Ref: British National Formulary, 1997.

QUESTION 14

A. TRUE B. TRUE C. TRUE D. FALSE E. TRUE

Bactericidal:
   Aminoglycosides, Penicillins, Cephalosporins,
   Co-trimoxazole, Isoniazid, Metronidazole, Vancomycin

Bacteriostatic:
   Erythromycin, Sulphonamides, Tetracyclines

Ref: W McCaughey, R S J Clarke, J P H Fee, W F M Wallace. Anaesthetic Physiology and Pharmacology, 1st ed. Churchill Livingstone, 1997.

QUESTION 15

A. FALSE B. FALSE C. TRUE D. TRUE E. TRUE

QUESTION 16

A. TRUE B. TRUE C. TRUE D. TRUE E. FALSE

Metronidazole is an antimicrobial drug with high activity against anaerobic bacteria and protozoa. It is also effective in the treatment of antibiotic-associated colitis (pseudomembranous colitis).

Ref: British National Formulary, 1997.

QUESTION 17

A. TRUE B. TRUE C. FALSE D. TRUE E. TRUE

Pulmonary fibrosis is not a recognised adverse effect of digoxin.

Ref: British National Formulary, 1997.

QUESTION 18

A. TRUE B. FALSE C. FALSE D. TRUE E. TRUE

Volatile anaesthetic agents produce a dose-related relaxation of uterine smooth muscle. Salbutamol and ritodrine (β_2-agonists) reduce uterine tone and are used to suppress premature labour. Uterine tone is not reduced by ketamine, the tendency being towards increased tone. Non-depolarising muscle relaxants have no effect on uterine smooth muscle.

Ref: W McCaughey, R S J Clarke, J P H Fee, W F M Wallace. Anaesthetic Physiology and Pharmacology, 1st ed. Churchill Livingstone, 1997.

QUESTION 19

A. TRUE B. TRUE C. TRUE D. TRUE E. TRUE

All are recognised side effects of the named drugs.

Drugs known to cause acute pancreatitis include:
    Azathioprine
    Cimetidine
    Frusemide
    Paracetamol
    Steroids
    Sulphonamides
    Tetracyclines
    Thiazides

Ref: British National Formulary, 1997.

QUESTION 20

A. TRUE B. FALSE C. TRUE D. TRUE E. FALSE

Helium is much less dense than nitrogen and in turbulent flow, as occurs in stridor and upper airway obstruction, a helium/oxygen mixtures decreases the work of breathing. Viscosities of helium and nitrogen are very similar. The thermal conductivity of helium is six times greater than that of nitrogen, making it a poorer insulator. Nitrogen at high pressure has a narcotic effect and this is the reason for the use of helium in deep diving.

Ref: R S Atkinson, G B Rushman, N J H Davies. Lee's Synopsis of Anaesthesia, 11th ed. Butterworth-Heinemann, 1993.

QUESTION 21

A. FALSE B. TRUE C. FALSE D. FALSE E. TRUE

Cyanosis occurs when the capillary blood has a reduced haemoglobin (not carbaminohaemoglobin) level over 5 g/dl. If the haemoglobin is normal it is usually detected at SaO_2 85-90% (PaO_2 6.7-8.0 kPa). Cyanosis is more readily provoked in the presence of polycythaemiA. If the haemoglobin is low it may not be detected however low the PaO_2. Cyanosis is unusual in carbon monoxide poisoning, because the colour of reduced haemoglobin is obscured by the cherry-red colour of carboxyhaemoglobin. Cyanosis does not occur in histotoxic hypoxia, because the blood gas content is normal. Cyanosis can also be detected when the methaemoglobin level is over 1.5 g/dl or the sulphaemoglobin level is over 0.5 g/dl.

Ref: R S Atkinson, G B Rushman, N J H Davies. Lee's Synopsis of Anaesthesia, 11th ed. Butterworth-Heinemann, 1993.

QUESTION 22

A. FALSE   B. FALSE   C. FALSE   D. TRUE   E. TRUE

The Valsalva manoeuvre is basically a forced expiration against a closed glottis. The patient blows a column of mercury up to 40 mmHg and maintains this pressure for 10 seconds. Blood pressure rises at the onset of straining because the increase in intrathoracic pressure is added to the pressure of the blood in the aorta. The blood pressure then falls because the high intrathoracic pressure decreases the venous return to the right atrium resulting in a decreased cardiac output. The fall in blood pressure and pulse pressure inhibits the baroreceptors, resulting in an increase in the peripheral resistance and a tachycardia. At the termination of the manoeuvre, intrathoracic pressure returns to normal, cardiac output is restored, but the peripheral vessels are still constricted. The blood pressure therefore rises above normal, and this stimulates the baroreceptors, causing bradycardia and a drop in blood pressure to normal. Approximately 20-40% of long-standing diabetics develop some degree of autonomic neuropathy. In patients with autonomic neuropathy of any cause, the heart rate changes are absent.

Ref: W F Ganong. Review of Medical Physiology, 18th ed. Lange, 1997.

QUESTION 23

A. FALSE   B. FALSE   C. TRUE   D. FALSE   E. TRUE

The baroreceptors (e.g. carotid sinus) consist of stretch receptors. Carotid and aortic bodies consist of chemoreceptors. The carotid body has a blood flow approximately forty times that of the brain (2000 ml/100g/min, compared to 54 ml/100g/min in the brain). Because of this enormous blood flow, the oxygen needs of the cells can be met by the dissolved oxygen alone. In anaemia and carbon monoxide poisoning, where the amount of dissolved oxygen in the blood remains normal, the receptors are not stimulated. The receptors of the carotid body are stimulated by an increase in $PaCO_2$, decrease in PaO_2, decrease in pH, vascular stasis (when the amount of oxygen delivered to the receptors per unit time is decreased) and cyanide (when tissue oxygen utilisation is prevented).

Ref: W F Ganong. Review of Medical Physiology, 18th ed. Lange, 1997.

QUESTION 24

A. TRUE   B. FALSE   C. TRUE   D. FALSE   E. TRUE

Thermoregulation is achieved through the autonomic nervous system by control of cutaneous vasoconstriction or vasodilatation. Thermoregulation maintains a steady body temperature in spite of fluctuations in the temperature of the environment. The components of the thermoregulation system form a network of negative feedback loops. The hypothalamus is the principal structure within the CNS in the co-ordination of thermoregulation. In neonates, brown fat is a useful source of heat production as shivering is not possible. It is found in the neck, the back and around the viscera. It is controlled by the sympathetic nervous system.

Ref: W F Ganong. Review of Medical Physiology, 18th ed. Lange, 1997.

QUESTION 25

A. TRUE B. TRUE C. TRUE D. FALSE E. FALSE

The hypothalamic temperature reflects core temperature. Sites shown to have a good correlation with hypothalamic temperature include the tympanic membrane, lower oesophagus, nasopharynx, bladder and the temperature of blood in the pulmonary artery.

Rectal temperature probes have slow response rates and may give rise to inaccurate readings due to the presence of faeces.

Ref: A R Aitkenhead, G Smith. Textbook of Anaesthesia, 3rd ed. Churchill Livingstone, 1996.

QUESTION 26

A. TRUE B. FALSE C. FALSE D. FALSE E. FALSE

There are gap junctions between muscle fibres, which provide low-resistance bridges for the spread of excitation. They permit cardiac muscle to function as if it were a syncytium. Like skeletal muscle, cardiac muscle contains myosin, actin, tropomyosin and troponin.

Each muscle fibre consists of a single nucleus, unlike skeletal muscle. Myocardial fibres have a resting membrane potential of approximately - 90 mV. At a heart rate of 75 beats per minute, the duration of the action potential is 250 ms.

Ref: W F Ganong. Review of Medical Physiology, 18th ed. Lange, 1997.

QUESTION 27

A. FALSE B. FALSE C. TRUE D. TRUE E. FALSE

The stellate and coeliac ganglia are sympathetic ganglia. The gasserian ganglion is the fifth cranial nerve ganglion.

Ref: W F Ganong. Review of Medical Physiology, 18th ed. Lange, 1997.

QUESTION 28

A. TRUE B. TRUE C. TRUE D. TRUE E. TRUE

Stellate ganglion block results in Horner's syndrome: ptosis, miosis, anhydrosis, enopthalmosis, dilated conjunctival vessels and nasal congestion.

Ref: R S Atkinson, G B Rushman, N J H Davies. Lee's Synopsis of Anaesthesia, 11th ed. Butterworth-Heinemann, 1993.

QUESTION 29

A. TRUE   B. FALSE   C. FALSE   D. FALSE   E. FALSE

	Pre-renal	ATN
Urine osmolality (mosmol/kg)	>450	<350
Urine sodium (mmol/l)	<10-20	>20-40
U:P osmolality	>2	<1.5
U:P creatinine	>40	<40
U:P urea	>8	<3

QUESTION 30

A. TRUE   B. FALSE   C. TRUE   D. FALSE   E. TRUE

A ventilation/perfusion (V/Q) ratio of less than 1.0 indicates that lung ventilation is impaired. This is the case where the alveoli are filled with pneumonia, pulmonary oedema and pulmonary contusion. With hypovolaemic shock and pulmonary embolus, lung perfusion is reduced relative to ventilation and the V/Q ratio is greater than 1.0.

QUESTION 31

A. TRUE   B. TRUE   C. FALSE   D. FALSE   E. FALSE

At birth, there is a marked decrease in pulmonary vascular resistance and an increase in systemic vascular resistance. There is right axis deviation due to a thicker right ventricle, but ventricular thickness is equal by 6 months and then becomes greater on the left-hand side.

The increased left atrial pressure as a result of increased blood flow closes the foramen ovale. It is the increase in PaO_2 which stimulates the closure of the ductus arteriosus. The haemoglobin at birth is approximately 18 g/dl, decreasing to approximately 10 g/dl by 3 months. Myelination of the nervous system is incomplete during the first year of life.

Ref: W F Ganong. Review of Medical Physiology, 18th ed. Lange, 1997.

QUESTION 32

A. FALSE   B. TRUE   C. TRUE   D. TRUE   E. TRUE

Pulmonary oedema is the extravascular accumulation of fluid within the lung. The Starling equation, describing the balance of hydrostatic and osmotic pressures, is fundamental to its understanding.

The following factors predispose to pulmonary oedema:-

- High pulmonary capillary pressure
(e.g. Left ventricular failure or mitral stenosis)

- Decreased oncotic pressure
(e.g. Hypoalbuminaemia)
- Increased capillary permeability
(e.g. ARDS, sepsis)
- Impairment of lymphatic drainage
(e.g. malignancy)
- Rapid lung expansion
(e.g. re-expansion of pneumothorax or relief of upper airway obstruction)

QUESTION 33

A. TRUE B. TRUE C. FALSE D. FALSE E. TRUE

Pulse pressure increases during exercise; systolic blood pressure rises, whereas diastolic pressure may remain unchanged or even decrease. There is a decrease in total peripheral resistance due to vasodilatation in exercising muscles. The respiratory quotient is the ratio of the volume of CO_2 produced to the volume of O_2 consumed per unit time. During exercise, the respiratory quotient may reach 2.0 because of hyperventilation and blowing off of CO_2 while contracting an O_2 debt. During exercise, there is little change in skin blood flow. Regional blood flow to the kidneys, liver and the gastrointestinal tract is reduced.

Ref: W F Ganong. Review of Medical Physiology, 18th ed. Lange, 1997.

QUESTION 34

A. TRUE B. FALSE C. FALSE D. TRUE E. TRUE

The A and B antigens are inherited in a autosomal dominant manner. An individual with type B blood may have inherited a B antigen from each parent or a B antigen from one parent and an O from the other.

Ref: W F Ganong. Review of Medical Physiology, 18th ed. Lange, 1997.

QUESTION 35

A. TRUE B. TRUE C. FALSE D. TRUE E. FALSE

PTH is a polypeptide chain containing 84 amino acid residues.

The actions of PTH include:-

- Increased tubular reabsorption of calcium
- Increased osteoclastic resorption of bone
- Increased calcium absorption from the intestine
- Increased synthesis of 1,25-dihydroxycholecalciferol
- Increased phosphate excretion in the urine

Plasma calcium, phosphate, alkaline phosphatase and PTH are all normal in osteoporosis.

Ref: W F Ganong. Review of Medical Physiology, 18th ed. Lange, 1997.

QUESTION   36

A. TRUE   B. FALSE   C. TRUE   D. TRUE   E. FALSE

The knee jerk reflex is an example of a monosynaptic reflex. The stimulus that initiates the reflex is stretch of the *quadriceps femoris* muscle on tapping the patellar tendon. The response is contraction of the muscle that is stretched. The sense organ within the muscle is the muscle spindle.

Ref: W F Ganong. Review of Medical Physiology, 18th ed. Lange, 1997.

QUESTION   37

A. TRUE   B. FALSE   C. FALSE   D. TRUE   E. FALSE

Smooth muscle, in contrast to skeletal and cardiac muscle, lacks visible cross-striations. It contains actin, myosin and tropomyosin but not troponin. Unlike skeletal muscle, smooth muscle comprises single nucleated cells. Like cardiac muscle, smooth muscle acts as a syncytium. The smooth muscle is innervated by the autonomic nervous system.

Ref: W F Ganong. Review of Medical Physiology, 18th ed. Lange, 1997.

QUESTION   38

A. TRUE   B. FALSE   C. FALSE   D. TRUE   E. FALSE

Skeletal muscle comprises multinucleated cells with no syncytial bridges between cells. The resting membrane potential is approximately - 90 mV. The action potential lasts between 2 to 4 ms. During contraction, the width of the A bands is constant, whereas the width of the I bands is reduced. During a complete tetanus, the tension developed is approximately 4 times that developed by an individual twitch contraction. Skeletal muscle is under somatic nervous control.

Ref: W F Ganong. Review of Medical Physiology, 18th ed. Lange, 1997.

QUESTION   39

A. FALSE   B. FALSE   C. TRUE   D. FALSE   E. FALSE

The ideal substance for determining glomerular filtration rate has to be freely filtered (i.e. not protein-bound and with a low molecular weight), not reabsorbed or secreted by the tubules, non-toxic, and not metabolised. Inulin, a polymer of fructose with a molecular weight of 5,200 meets these criteria.

Ref: W F Ganong. Review of Medical Physiology, 18th ed. Lange, 1997.

QUESTION 40

A. TRUE   B. TRUE   C. FALSE   D. TRUE   E. TRUE

'Dumping' of food into the jejunum results in hyperglycaemia, which is followed by insulin-induced hypoglycaemia. Protein digestion is not affected. Iron deficiency anaemia may occur due to poor absorption. Megaloblastic anaemia may occur due to either folate deficiency (as a result of poor intake) or Vitamin B_{12} deficiency (if a source of intrinsic factor necessary for Vitamin B_{12} absorption is lost).

QUESTION 41

A. TRUE   B. TRUE   C. TRUE   D. TRUE   E. TRUE

Exponential relationships can also be expressed in terms of half-lives or time constants. A time constant is the time at which the process would have been completed had the initial rate of change continued. After 1 time constant 36.8% of the original value remains, after 2 time constants 13.5% and after 3 time constants 5%. One half-life is equal to 0.698 of the time constant.

QUESTION 42

A. FALSE   B. FALSE   C. FALSE   D. FALSE   E. FALSE

The Bain circuit is the coaxial version of the Mapleson D system. Fresh gas flow (FGF) is supplied through a narrow inner tube. The patient's expired gases pass through the outer tube and are vented to atmosphere. This system is inefficient during spontaneous breathing but efficient during controlled ventilation. A FGF rate of between two to three times minute volume (200–250 ml/kg/min) may be required during spontaneous ventilation to prevent rebreathing. FGF of between 70 and 80 ml/kg/min is required during controlled ventilation to prevent rebreathing.

The Lack circuit is the coaxial version of the Mapleson A system. The outer tube supplies inspired gas from the reservoir bag and the patient exhales through the inner tube. This system is inefficient during controlled ventilation but efficient during spontaneous breathing. During controlled ventilation, the FGF rate must be at least three times alveolar minute volume to prevent rebreathing. If the system is functioning correctly and no leaks are present, a FGF rate equal to the patient's alveolar minute ventilation is sufficient to prevent rebreathing. In practice, a higher FGF rate (equal to the minute volume) is selected to compensate for leaks. Unlike the Bain circuit, the Lack circuit does not permit the use of ventilators to provide controlled ventilation.

Ref: A R Aitkenhead, G Smith. Textbook of Anaesthesia, 3rd ed. Churchill Livingstone, 1996.

QUESTION 43

A. FALSE   B. TRUE   C. FALSE   D. FALSE   E. FALSE

When the bundle of His conducts normally but one of the bundle branches is blocked, the PR interval is normal but the QRS complex is widened. Bundle branch block does not significantly impair cardiac function, and of itself is not responsible for any symptoms the patient may have. RBBB often indicates problems in the right side of the heart, but RBBB patterns with a normal duration of the QRS complex are quite common in healthy people. LBBB is always an indication of heart disease.

When the PR interval lengthens progressively with each beat, and then a P wave fails to conduct, the Wenckebach block (Mobitz type I) is present. Pacing is not usually considered necessary in an asymptomatic patient with Mobitz type I block.

In normal ECGs the T wave is always inverted in VR, but is usually upright in all other leads. In young people the R-R interval is reduced (heart rate is increased) during inspiration and this is called sinus arrhythmia. It is lost in autonomic neuropathy.

Ref: J R Hampton. The ECG in Practice, 1st ed. Churchill Livingstone, 1986.

QUESTION 44

A. FALSE B. FALSE C. TRUE D. FALSE E. TRUE

ECG changes occur late and may show right heart strain and arrhythmias. Cyanosis also occurs late, so pulse oximetry will not provide an early detection of air embolus. Capnography provides an early detection of air embolus by a sudden drop in the end-tidal CO_2 reading. Auscultation with the stethoscope is insensitive and the classical 'millwheel' murmur occurs late. Doppler ultrasound is a very sensitive method for the detection of air embolus (0.5 ml).

Ref: A R Aitkenhead, G Smith. Textbook of Anaesthesia, 3rd ed. Churchill Livingstone, 1996.

QUESTION 45

A. TRUE B. FALSE C. TRUE D. FALSE E. FALSE

Pressure-volume loops can be used for measurement of compliance and work of breathing. Compliance is the change in lung volume per unit change in airway pressure. Work is defined in terms of mass and distance moved which, for the lung, is expressed as volume and pressure.

FRC can be measured by one of three methods: helium dilution, body plethysmograph and nitrogen washout.

Measurement of airway resistance requires the measurement of flow. The simplest method relies upon simultaneous measurement of airflow, and the mouth-pleural pressure gradient. The subject breathes or is ventilated through a pneumotachograph to give a measure of air flow which may be integrated to derive tidal volume. Pleural pressure is obtained from oesophageal pressure.

Closing volume can be measured by the analysis of the single-breath nitrogen curves.

Ref: W S Nimmo, G Smith. Anaesthesia, 2nd ed. Blackwell, 1994.

QUESTION 46

A. FALSE B. FALSE C. TRUE D. FALSE E. FALSE

Helium and argon do not support combustion and are non-flammable. Nitrous oxide supports combustion, although it is not flammable. Carbon dioxide does not support combustion and is used in fire extinquishers. Modern volatile anaesthetic agents (halothane, enflurane, isoflurane, desflurane and sevoflurane) do not support combustion and in clinical concentrations are non-flammable.

Ref: A R Aitkenhead, G Smith. Textbook of Anaesthesia, 3rd ed. Churchill Livingstone, 1996.

QUESTION 47

A. FALSE B. FALSE C. TRUE D. TRUE E. FALSE

Laminar flow is governed by Poiseuille's law:-
- Flow is proportional to the driving pressure
- Flow is proportional to the radius to the power of 4
- Flow is inversely related to the viscosity of fluid
- Flow is inversely related to the length of the tube

Note the critical role of the tube radius: for laminar flow, halving the radius decreases the flow 16-fold for the same driving pressure. This fact is of great importance in paediatric practice and also provides part of the explanation for the rapid decompensation of patients with progressive airway narrowing.

The relationship for turbulent flow is more complex (and depends on which book you read) but may be stated as:-
- Flow is proportional to the square root of the driving pressure
- Flow is proportional to the square of the radius
- Flow is inversely related to the square root of the density of fluid

The likelihood of laminar or turbulent flow may be predicted from Reynolds' number (Re). This is a dimensionless number derived from the product of the diameter, velocity and density, divided by the viscosity.

Values for Re in excess of 2,000 are likely to result in turbulent flow and less than 1,000 in laminar flow.

Ref: W S Nimmo, G Smith. Anaesthesia, 2nd ed. Blackwell, 1994.

QUESTION 48

A. FALSE B. TRUE C. TRUE D. FALSE E. TRUE

	Viscosity	Density
Air	18.2	1.196
Nitrogen	17.6	1.165
Oxygen	20.4	1.331
Carbon dioxide	14.7	1.831
Nitrous oxide	14.6	1.831
Helium	19.6	0.166

70% nitrous oxide in oxygen is less viscous but more dense than air. Thus turbulent flow is more likely to occur in anaesthetised patients, which may be relevant in patients with an increased airway resistance who are allowed to breathe spontaneously.

Helium has a very low density. In upper airway obstruction, flow is inevitably turbulent. The extent of turbulent flow may be reduced by reducing gas density. Clinically, it may be beneficial to administer oxygen-enriched helium rather than oxygen alone. It should be noted, however, that helium has a high viscosity and therefore confers no advantage in laminar flow conditions.

Carbon dioxide and nitrous oxide have very similar viscosity and density and their flowmeters are therefore interchangeable. This is however, not recommended in practice! The viscosity of a gas increases with increase in temperature, whereas the viscosity of a liquid decreases with increase in temperature.

Ref: W S Nimmo, G Smith. Anaesthesia, 2nd ed. Blackwell, 1994.

QUESTION 49

A. FALSE B. TRUE C. TRUE D. FALSE E. TRUE

Active scavenging systems employ some device to generate a negative pressure within the system to expel the waste gases to the outside atmosphere. This may be a vacuum pump or a Venturi system.

In a passive scavenging system, gas movement is generated by the patient. Such a system consists of a simple network of tubing in which the resistance to flow does not exceed 50 Pa (0.5 cmH$_2$O) at 30 l/min. A reservoir bag is needed to accommodate high flows during expiration. A safety block provides positive and negative pressure relief which is set to blow off at pressures outside the -50 to 1,000 Pa (-0.5 to 10 cmH$_2$O) range. A discharge point consisting of a T-termination with downward angled ends is commonly used. Each scavenging system should have a separate external terminal to prevent gases being vented into adjacent locations. Negative pressures may be generated by certain wind conditions at the external terminal. The relief valve at -50 Pa limits this.

Ref: T M Craft, P M Upton. Key Topics in Anaesthesia, 1st ed. BIOS Scientific Publishers, 1992.

QUESTION 50

A. FALSE B. FALSE C. FALSE D. TRUE E. FALSE

During intense neuromuscular stimulation, the response to single twitch, train-of-four (ToF) and tetanic stimuli are all zero. The post-tetanic count (PTC) was designed to be used in this circumstance, and it applies the post-tetanic facilitation principle. It consists of a 5-second, 50-Hz tetanus followed, 3 seconds later, by at least 20 stimulations delivered at 1 Hz. The number of detectable twitches is inversely related to the degree of blockade. If 12-15 post-tetanic twitches are observed, reappearance of a response to ToF stimulation is imminent. Because tetanic stimulation may facilitate further tetanic responses, it is recommended not to apply PTC more often than every 5 minutes.

70-80% of receptors have to be occupied by neuromuscular blocking drug before the response to nerve stimulation is affected. Accordingly, during recovery from neuromuscular blockade even with normal inspiratory force, vital capacity, protrusion of the tongue and sustained head lift for 5 seconds, 70-80% of all receptors can still be occupied by the neuromuscular blocker. At a time when both clinical criteria and response to nerve stimulation indicate sufficient recovery of neuromuscular function, about 70% of receptors may still be occupied by the neuromuscular blocking agent.

ToF-Watch and ToF-Guard use acceleromyography for monitoring neuromuscular block. These systems contain a piezoelectric ceramic wafer with electrodes on both sides. Acceleromyography is based on Newton's second law: *force = mass × acceleration*. Thus, if the mass is constant, acceleration is directly proportional to force of contraction.

Ref: T E J Healy, P J Cohen. Wylie and Churchill-Davidson's A Practice of Anaesthesia, 6th ed. Edward Arnold, 1995.

QUESTION 51

A. TRUE B. TRUE C. TRUE D. FALSE E. TRUE

When a volatile liquid is in contact with its vapour in a closed container, the vapour concentration increases because many more molecules escape from the liquid than rejoin it. However, a condition is reached at which these processes are equally frequent and the system reaches equilibrium. The vapour is then fully saturated and exerts a characteristic partial pressure at the prevailing temperature.

The SVP increases with temperature according to a complex (Antoine) equation. For instance, the SVP of halothane at $21°C$ is 32.4 kPa, which at standard barometric pressure corresponds to a concentration of $32.4/101.3 × 100 = 32\%$. This is the highest attainable concentration under these conditions of temperature and pressure.

If the liquid is heated, the vapour pressure rises until ultimately it reaches atmospheric pressure, the liquid boils and the gas phase consists of 100% vapour. Clearly, this temperature (the boiling point) is dependent upon the atmospheric pressure and therefore upon altitude.

At high altitude, the boiling point is reduced, and the SVP is a greater proportion of the total pressure; thus, the concentration of saturated gas is increased. At an altitude of 1,000 metres above sea level, the atmospheric pressure is approximately 90 kPa, and therefore a saturated halothane vapour contains 32.4/90 × 100 = 36%.

The SVP is independent of the ambient pressure, but increases with increasing temperature.

The boiling point is the temperature at which its SVP becomes equal to the ambient pressure.

Latent heat of vaporisation is the energy required to change a liquid to vapour at a constant temperature. It is defined at a specified temperature as it decreases as the temperature increases. When the temperature reaches the critical temperature the energy required to vaporise the liquid is zero (vaporisation occurs spontaneously) and above this temperature the substance cannot exist as a liquid.

Ref: W S Nimmo, G Smith. Anaesthesia, 2nd ed. Blackwell, 1994.

QUESTION 52

A. FALSE B. TRUE C. FALSE D. TRUE E. FALSE

The critical temperature of a substance is the temperature above which that substance cannot be liquefied by pressure, irrespective of the magnitude of that pressure.

Critical temperature (°C)

Oxygen	–118
Entonox	–5.5
Air	–141

Thus, at room temperature, cylinders of these substances all contain gases.

In contrast, the critical temperature of carbon dioxide is 31°C (critical pressure 73.8 bar) and that of nitrous oxide 36.4°C (critical pressure 72.5 bar). At pressures higher than their critical pressures, these substances contain a mixture of gas and liquid.

Ref: A R Aitkenhead, G Smith. Textbook of Anaesthesia, 3rd ed. Churchill Livingstone, 1996.

QUESTION 53

A. TRUE B. TRUE C. FALSE D. FALSE E. FALSE

The Rotameter consists of a bobbin in a vertical, tapered glass tube, up which a gas is passed. With increasing flow the bobbin is displaced upwards. As the bobbin moves upwards, the space around it increases in width so that a greater gas flow is required to support the bobbin itself.

At low flow rates, the width of the annulus is small so that it behaves like a tube through which gas flows at low velocity with a laminar profile. Here, the pressure drop across the annulus (which provides the force to support the bobbin) is proportional to the flow rate, and depends upon the gas viscosity.

At high flow rates, the gap between bobbin and glass wall is much wider, and the annulus behaves like an orifice. Flow becomes turbulent and the upward force on the bobbin is now proportional to the square of the flow rate. Gas density is more important than viscosity.

Over a wide range of flow rates, calibration of the flowmeter is dependent upon both viscosity and density.

	Viscosity	Density
Air	18.2	1.196
Oxygen	20.4	1.331
Carbon dioxide	14.7	1.831
Nitrous oxide	14.6	1.831

If passed through identical flowmeters at the same rates, carbon dioxide and nitrous oxide yield very similar readings.

Ref: W S Nimmo, G Smith. Anaesthesia, 2nd ed. Blackwell, 1994.

QUESTION 54

A. TRUE B. TRUE C. TRUE D. TRUE E. FALSE

A circle system is composed of two unidirectional valves (inspiratory and expiratory), an over-flow valve, a reservoir bag, a soda-lime canister and a fresh gas inlet, all connected by tubing. Although numerous arrangements of the components are possible, maximal efficiency can be achieved by the following:-

- The fresh gas inlet is positioned in the inspired gas stream proximal to the inspiratory valve ensuring maximum inspired concentration of oxygen and anaesthetic gases.
- Expired gas is vented via the overflow valve from the circuit upstream of the soda lime, to conserve the soda-lime.
- The soda-lime is placed downstream of the overflow valve but before the fresh gas inlet. This has the combined effect of reducing respiratory resistance and because of the low flow rate allows adequate time for absorption.
- The reservoir bag is positioned upstream of the soda-lime.

Ref: W S Nimmo, G Smith. Anaesthesia, 2nd ed. Blackwell, 1994.

QUESTION 55

A. FALSE   B. FALSE   C. FALSE   D. TRUE   E. TRUE

If current is delivered to a whole nerve trunk, and if its intensity is too low for threshold to be reached in any of the nerve fibres, no action potential will be propagated. As current is further increased, all nerve fibres are sufficiently depolarised to initiate an action potential. Increasing the stimulus intensity would not further increase the number of action potentials. The electrical stimulus applied is usually 25% above that necessary for a maximal response. For this reason, the stimulus is said to be supramaximal. This is up to 50 mA for surface electrode and up to 10 mA for needle electrode.

Once an action potential has been generated, the nerve is insensitive to further stimulation for a certain interval, the refractory period, which is usually 1-2 ms. If the duration of the electrical stimulus is greater than the refractory period, another action potential may be triggered or the muscle may be stimulated directly. If, however, the stimulus duration is too short, there might be insufficient time for the nerve membrane to reach threshold. The optimum pulse duration is 0.2 ms. The impulse should be monophasic and rectangular (i.e. a square wave).

Most stimulators deliver tetanic stimulations at a frequency of 50 Hz for 5 seconds. For a 50 Hz, 5 second tetanus, post-tetanic potentiation persists for at least 1-2 minutes. Train-of-four (ToF) stimulation is the most popular mode of stimulation for clinical monitoring of neuromuscular function. It consists of four pulses delivered every 0.5 seconds (2 Hz). With such a small number of stimuli delivered, there is no post-tetanic potentiation, and the neuromuscular junction recovers rapidly, within 10-12 seconds. After this interval, ToF stimulation can be reapplied.

Ref: T E J Healy, P J Cohen. Wylie and Churchill-Davidson's A Practice of Anaesthesia, 6th ed. Edward Arnold, 1995.

QUESTION 56

A. FALSE   B. TRUE   C. FALSE   D. TRUE   E. TRUE

Abductor pollicis brevis and *opponens pollicis* are supplied by the median nerve. *Adductor pollicis* is supplied by the ulnar nerve. *Orbicularis oculi* is supplied by the facial nerve. Muscles in the anterior aspect of the lower limb (e.g. *tibialis anterior*) are supplied by the common peroneal nerve causing dorsiflexion of the foot. The muscles of the posterior aspect of the lower limb are supplied by the tibial nerve causing plantar flexion of the foot.

The *orbicularis oculi* response to facial nerve stimulation reflects the extent of neuromuscular blockade of the diaphragm better than does the response of the *adductor pollicis* to ulnar nerve stimulation.

QUESTION 57

A. FALSE   B. FALSE   C. TRUE   D. FALSE   E. FALSE

Different muscles exhibit different sensitivities to neuromuscular blocking drugs. For example, under the same stimulation conditions, the diaphragm is less sensitive than the *tibialis anterior* muscle. For clinical relaxation, the diaphragm requires 90% receptor occupancy and *adductor pollicis* 70%, whereas the *tibialis anterior* needs only 20%. *Adductor pollicis* may thus still be paralysed, even after the patient has resumed normal respiration. This is significant, because *adductor pollicis* is often used for monitoring.

Sensitivities of different muscle groups to non-depolarising neuromuscular blocker in descending order:-

> *Tibialis anterior*
> *Geniohyoid*
> *Masseter*
> *Adductor pollicis*
> Abdominal muscles
> Diaphragm
> *Orbicularis oculi*
> Laryngeal adductors

Stimulation of the ulnar nerve causes adduction of the thumb (*adductor pollicis*). Stimulation of the common peroneal nerve causes dorsiflexion of the foot. It is stimulation of the posterior tibial nerve that causes planter flexion.

Ref: T E J Healy, P J Cohen. Wylie and Churchill-Davidson's A Practice of Anaesthesia, 6th ed. Edward Arnold, 1995.

QUESTION 58

A. TRUE   B. TRUE   C. TRUE   D. TRUE   E. TRUE

The response to non-depolarising neuromuscular blocker is different in different muscles, both in terms of onset and intensity of blockade. Onset of neuromuscular block is more rapid at the diaphragm and larynx than at the *adductor pollicis*. Neuromuscular blockers produce less intense block at the *orbicularis oculi* than the *adductor pollicis*. Paradoxically, onset of blockade is faster at the *orbicularis oculi*. This difference is probably related to the differences in muscle blood flow and distance to the central circulation between centrally located and peripheral muscle.

The train-of-four (ToF) technique uses four stimuli given at 0.5 s intervals (2 Hz). The fourth evoked response is eliminated at about 75% depression of the control, the third at 80% and the second at 90%. Absence of all four indicates complete block. A T4/T1 ratio >75% is equivalent to being able to raise the head from the pillow, have normal respiratory function tests, the ability to cough properly, to open the eyes and protrude the tongue on command.

The visual and tactile assessment of residual blockade is often difficult. Double-burst stimulation (DBS) is more sensitive than ToF for manual detection of small degrees of non–depolarising block. Two short 50 Hz bursts, separated by 750 ms, each burst containing three stimuli are used. During partial neuromuscular block, the response to the second burst is less than that of the first, so fade is present. The magnitude of this fade is similar to ToF fade. However, human senses can detect DBS fade better. Trained observers are often unable to detect fade when the ToF ratio is as low as 0.2-0.3. When DBS is used, determination of fade is possible when the ToF ratio is 0.5-0.6 or less.

Ref: W S Nimmo, G Smith. Anaesthesia, 2nd ed. Blackwell, 1994.

QUESTION 59

A. TRUE B. FALSE C. TRUE D. TRUE E. FALSE

Gases whose molecules contain two dissimilar atoms or more than two atoms absorb radiation in the infrared region of the spectrum. Anaesthetic agents, especially nitrous oxide, interfere with the measurement of CO_2 by infrared absorption spectroscopy. $ETCO_2$ is approximately 0.5 kPa less than $PaCO_2$ in normal lungs. The $ETCO_2$ reading falls with emboli (air, blood or fat) because the embolised area does not exchange CO_2 into alveolar gas. The reading also falls in hypotension and a decreased cardiac output.

Ref: R S Atkinson, G B Rushman, N J H Davies. Lee's Synopsis of Anaesthesia, 11th ed. Butterworth-Heinemann, 1993.

QUESTION 60

A. TRUE B. FALSE C. FALSE D. TRUE E. FALSE

Since pulse oximeters are dual-wavelength devices, the presence of haemoglobin species other than reduced Hb and O_2Hb must therefore result in erroneous readings. An increasing concentration of carboxyhaemoglobin makes the pulse oximeter reading tend towards 100%. Pulse oximetry has been reported to be accurate in patients with haemoglobin S disease. It should be noted that patients with Sickle cell disease show a shift to the right of the oxy-haemoglobin dissociation curve, and therefore at any given PaO_2 value the oxygen saturation will be lower than expected. Bilirubin causes no significant effect on pulse oximetry. Pulse oximeters tend to underestimate actual oxygen saturation with significant anaemia. Polycythaemia has no apparent effect upon pulse oximetry reading.

Ref: R D Miller. Anesthesia, 4th ed. Churchill Livingstone, 1994.

NOTES

NOTES

NOTES

NOTES

QBase Anaesthesia on CD-ROM

SYSTEM REQUIREMENTS

An IBM compatible PC with a minimum 80386 processor and 4Mb of RAM VGA Monitor set up to display at least 256 colours.
CD-ROM drive
Windows 3.1 or higher with Microsoft compatible mouse
The display setting of your computer must be set to display "SMALL FONTS".
See Windows manuals for further instructions on how to do this.

INSTALLATION INSTRUCTIONS

The program will install the appropriate files onto your hard drive. It requires the QBase CD-ROM to be installed in the D:\drive.

In order to run to run QBase the CD-ROM must be in the drive.

Print Readme.txt and Helpfile.txt on the CD-ROM for fuller instructions and user manual

WINDOWS 95/98

1. Insert the QBase CD-ROM into drive **D:**
2. From the **Start Menu,** select the RUN **option**
3. Type **D:\setup.exe and press enter or return**
4. **Follow the Full Installation** option and accept the default directory for installation of QBase. The installation program creates a folder called **QBase** containing the program icon and another called **Exams** into which you can save previous exam attempts.
5. To run QBase double click the **QBase** icon in the QBase folder. From windows Explorer double click the **QBase.exe** file in the QBase folder.

WINDOWS 3.1/WINDOWS FOR WORKGROUPS 3.11

1. Insert the QBase CD-ROM into the drive D:
2. From the **File Menu,** select the **RUN option**
3. Type **D:\setup.exe and press enter or return**
4. Follow the instructions given by the installation program. Select the **Full Installation** option and accept the default directory for installation of QBase

   The Installation program creates a program window and directory called **QBase** containing the program icon. It also creates a directory called **Exams** into which you can save previous attempts.
5. To run QBase double click on the **QBase** icon in the QBase program. From File Manager double click the **QBase.exe** file in the QBase directory.